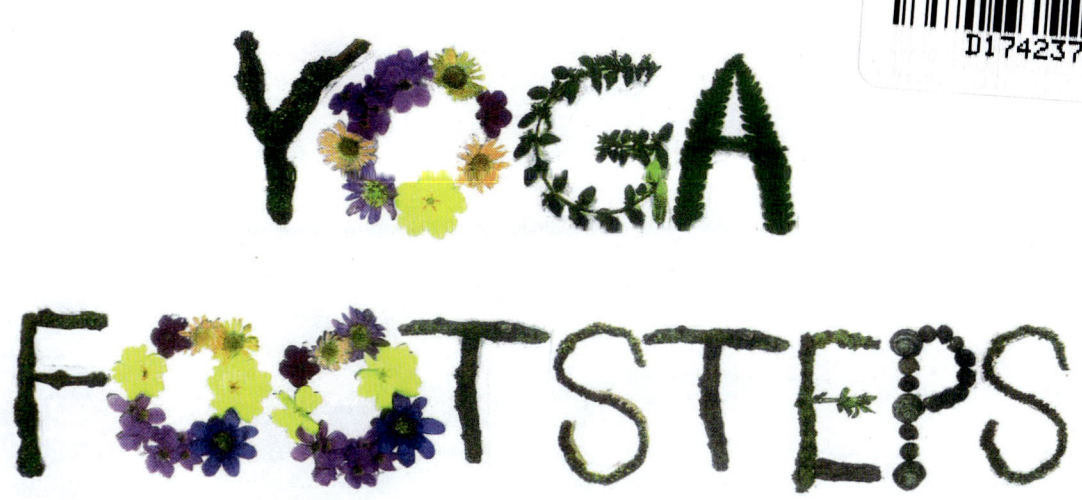

YOGA FOOTSTEPS

Written and Illustrated
by Vani Devi

ISBN 978-0-9524781-2-6

The writer/publisher of this book does not accept responsibility for any accident, injury or problem caused by practising the breath work, meditations or postures in this book. Not all postures and practices are appropriate for all people. It is your responsibility to know your body and its limitations and to choose suitable practices. Please read the 'Cautions and Health Issues' before commencing your practice and consult a medical practitioner if necessary.

Edited by Hazel Anderson and Clair Harwood
Printed and bound by Halstan Printing Group, HP6 6HJ. UK.

Published by Kool Kat Publications, 1 Dene Way, Newbury, Berks, RG14 2JL

Tel: 00 44 (0)1635 45300
E-mail: koolkatpub@hotmail.com
www.koolkatpublications.co.uk

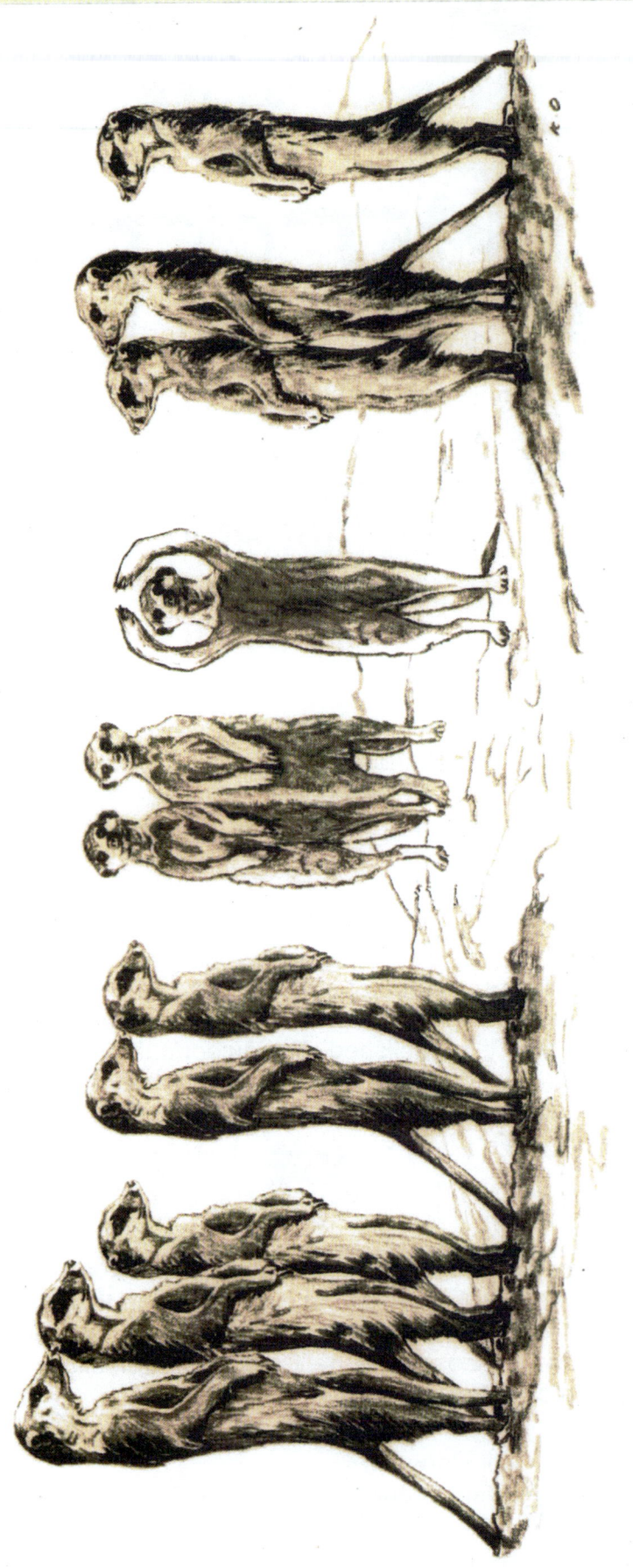

Meerkat Yoga Class

Contents

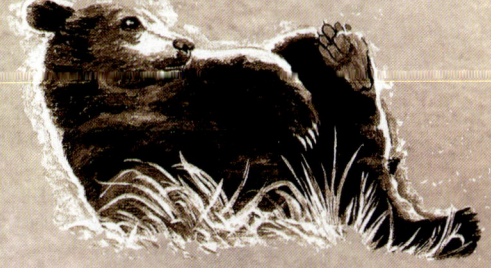

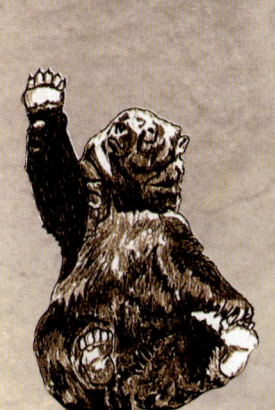

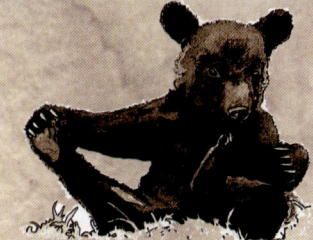

The Preface

After completing my last book, **Yoga Sequences Companion** (2011), I said I wasn't going to write any more books. Inevitably, the ideas kept coming from various sources and some were too good to leave floating in outer space. I find I forget about ideas I don't illustrate and write up and I can't read my writing if I just make notes. This is a very fertile time in the world of Yoga. The Internet may have negative impacts in some areas of existence but for yoga and spirituality it has been a great blessing. However, involvement with it has to be carefully monitored. Sitting for hours doing research is unhealthy and many contradictions are found in the assembled information.

I have named the sources of ideas whenever possible. Nearly all come from workshops or videos and from Yoga or Chi Gong backgrounds. An exception is the Native American Planting Chant. I have included this because it connects people to nature and makes them happy. I taught a seated version in an old people's home and they loved it so much, we did it every week. There were three people of 104 in the class and everybody had broad smiles on their faces when we finished it. However, in another class a young man got embarrassed and said, 'I can't do that,' and in my first U3A class (University of the Third Age), a lady walked out when we did it. Another lady said, 'That's the most bizarre thing I have ever done,' but she said it in an appreciative way.

As in my previous yoga books, this one is written with the average person in mind. It is more emotional than academic. The more intense, esoteric practices of the ancient yogis need to be taught by a Master in a quiet, appropriate environment. They are not compatible with the everyday existence of most people in the world today. The wise words of Krishnamacharya[1] are relevant here. He said, *'It is not for the individual to adapt her/himself to Yoga, rather for yoga to adapt itself to the individual.'* It is because yoga is so busy adapting to our fast-changing circumstances, via the minds of the ever-growing band of yoga teachers, that so many powerful ideas are manifesting.

The title of the book, Yoga Footsteps, implies a beginning and a journey. The footprints on the cover had to be from Indian feet, so I asked my Indian friend and pupil, who had been a lodger in my house for about five years, to tread in some brown paint for me.

I have included a few pages with essential information from previous books. This is for the benefit of newcomers to yoga. I consider an understanding of **The Full Yogic Breath** and **The Sympathetic and Parasympathetic Nervous Systems** to be the best life-enhancing tools on the planet.

My pupils are more involved in this book than in previous ones. One, who was a speech therapist, did the research on **Aphantasia** and helped me explain the vocalisation of OM in the **Heart Opening Sequence**. Another, a doctor who wished to remain anonymous, wrote about the arches of the feet after the **Tone Your Arches** sequence. A private pupil, who has been coming to me for over two years, wrote the page about **Electromagnetic Energy**. She has emphysema and CPOD and I have learnt as much from her as she has learnt from me. Another, who is interested in Egyptology, told me about the hands coming from the sun's rays for the **Gayatri Mudra Sequence**. She brought me the photographs I made the sketches from and added the information about them. Another brought me photos of her dogs doing doggy postures.

Those hoping for advanced postures in this book will be disappointed. Since I turned 70, in March 2014, my classes have gradually become gentler and less physically demanding. I still teach some postures I can no longer do myself but, inevitably, I teach less advanced posture work. That doesn't mean it is less beneficial.

I would like to thank all my pupils for their encouragement and participation in my classes. They are my guinea pigs, the ones I try out all my new ideas with, and without them this book would not have been written. Special thanks must go to my proof reader Rachel Tapping and my two editors, Hazel Anderson and Clair Harwood, also to Elisa Burato M.Ost., James Boag and Bob Camp for their contributions. There are many other people I would like to thank. Their names are too numerous to mention.

My observation is that the many different schools of yoga, all over the world, are contributing to opening people's minds and hearts. My wish is that the human hearts on this planet are given the opportunity to open to their full, glorious potential.

My background information

I studied the guitar and singing at the Guildhall School of Music in the 1960s. Kate Oppel (née Stuckey) is my married name. My first career was teaching the guitar in schools and as a singer/guitarist. In my early forties, I had a consultation with a Harley Street speech therapist about a problem that developed at the age of ten. The therapist advised me, 'I can't do anything for you but I suggest you take up yoga'. About two years later I finally made it to a local class and yoga has subsequently become an essential part of my life.

---

1. Krishnamacharya (1888-1989) taught yoga in the Mysore Palace in southern India. Three of his disciples went on to develop very different styles of posture work. They are P. Jois (Astanga Vinyasa Yoga), his son T. K. V. Desikkachar (aYs) and B. K. S. Iyengar (Iyengar Yoga).

I took the Sivananda Yoga Teachers Training Course in the Bahamas in 1998. I was given my spiritual name there. Vani Devi means Goddess of Speech and Song. I started teaching straight away in local village halls and The Pinnacle Leisure Centre (now Nuffield Health) in Newbury. In 2001, I started teaching people whose lives have been disrupted by mental health problems in Reading. In the same year, I took the Sivananda Advanced Course in Canada. I have taught young offenders in Reading Prison and patients in a psychiatric hospital in Reading and am still teaching mentally and physically vulnerable people.

In 2004, I took a Sadhana Intensive in the Himalayas and again in France in 2005 and 2007. This course involves studying the *Hatha Yoga Pradipika* and going deeper into the practice of *Pranayama* (exploring the potential of the breath). I feel it is the energy that I generated during these courses that facilitated my book writing.

I am very fortunate to be living in an area which is overflowing with yogic activity. I have had the opportunity to explore different styles of posture work, ranging from Dru to Iyengar. Many British Wheel of Yoga Congresses and workshops have also been catalytic.

As I teach open, mixed ability classes, it has been necessary to develop different ways of practising the postures. Also, as yoga teaching is usually taught in England and other countries in weekly classes or in terms, the class routine becomes part of our pupil's lives. I have met teachers who have been teaching the same pupils for 25 and 40 years on this basis. Although repetition is an essential part of yoga practice, innovation is necessary to keep the lessons interesting and develop potential.

Observations

I have spoken to yoga teachers about weekly lesson planning and it appears to be a major challenge for some. I know I'm more relaxed when I have worked out mine. It helps to have a few lesson plans that you can repeat about three times a year. It takes the pressure off. I have included a whole **So Hum Class** in this book and that is one of those classes. Other classes I repeat are the basic **Sivananda Class**, **Restorative**, **Gym Ball**, a **Yin and Yang** class and recently a **Circling Class**. I developed the latter by including the two circling sequences in this book. I start with **Figure of Eight Breathing** and conclude with the **Swimming Dragon** and **Swimming Dragon Meditation**, both from my last book. One of my pupils, who is a kinesiologist, said it was her favourite class.

Other books self-published by the Author
Blues Guitar, Play it your Way (Kate Oppel) (1994)   ISBN 0-9524781-02
Yoga Sequences (2003)   ISBN 0-9524781-0
Yoga Sequences Book 2 (2007)   ISBN 0-9524781-8-8
Yoga Expanded and Simplified (2009)   ISBN 978-0-9524781-4-0
Yoga Sequences Companion: A compilation of   ISBN 978-0-9524781-7-1
previous publications and new material (2011)
2nd Edition (2015) Published by **Yoga Words**, an   ISBN 978-1-906756-35-2
imprint of Pinter and Martin Ltd, London, SW2 1PS
Reprint (2017)

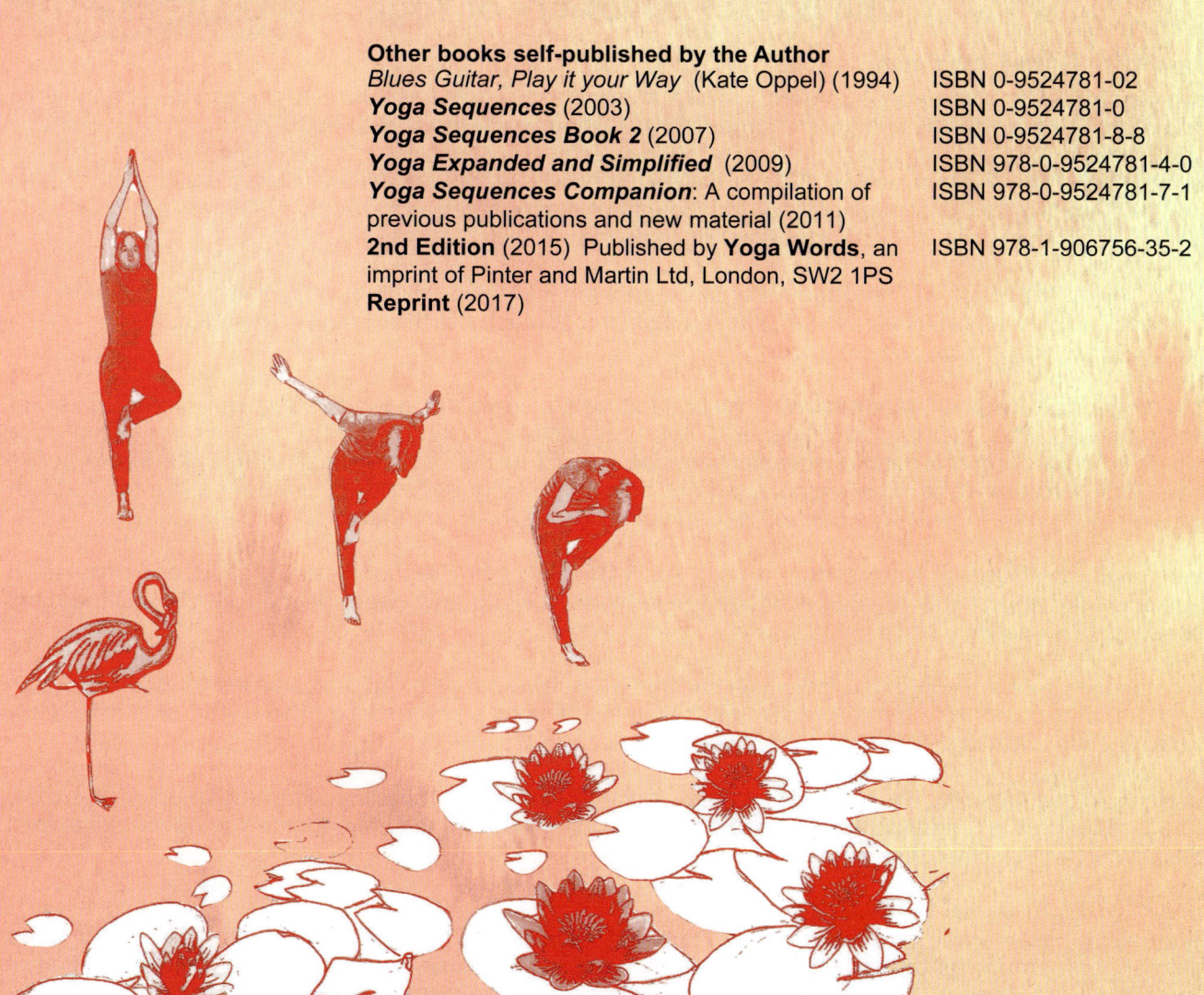

Foreword

I am delighted to have this opportunity to write the foreword to Vani Devi's new book on yoga.

Vani Devi is a highly creative person being not only a teacher of yoga and meditation, but also a musician, artist and writer. In an age where everyone seems to be trying to carve out a yoga niche, Vani Devi stands for diversity, creativity and inclusion in her approach to yoga.

In this book, you will find lovely, imaginative practices and sequences, using breath, sound and visualisation. Vani Devi's yoga tool box has grown large and varied over decades of teaching and there is something for everyone here. Whether you love to practise yoga, or teach and want some superb ideas to inspire your lessons, this book is for you.

Got students in a chair? No problem: Vani Devi has the answer. Having trouble weaving a theme through your classes? Vani Devi has a wealth of visualisations, imagery and practices to enrich your teaching. Practising at home? Vani Devi transcends most home practice books with the breadth and diversity of her grasp of the yoga tradition, while always honouring it.

I wish I'd had this book when I was starting out on my yoga journey. There is something for everyone and sections which blend science with yoga theory provide some "wow" moments.

Vani Devi is a familiar face at British Wheel of Yoga Congresses and events and I wish her great success in reaching the widest possible audience with this excellent book.

Paul Fox, Chair of BWY
April 2017

The Basic Framework of Yoga

The Four Paths of Yoga
Lord Krishna, who lived about 2,000BC, spoke about these four paths. His teachings were transmitted orally for many generations and finally narrated in the **Bhagavad Gita** (c.600-500BC).

Karma Yoga, the Yoga of action. This is selfless service towards our fellow human beings, the Planet Earth and the Higher Consciousness with no thought of personal reward. Deeds, not words are important. The good and bad usage of words corresponds to deeds.

Bhakti Yoga, the Yoga of Devotion. This is an emotional longing for involvement with the cosmos and Higher Consciousness. Words are not used to justify the emotion but to express it in singing and chanting, ceremony, ritual and story telling.

Raja Yoga, the Yoga of Meditation. This is mind control with the goal of achieving higher states of consciousness. The asanas and contents of this book belong to this path. The body is controlled as a prelude to controlling the mind. Particular attention is paid to the movement of prana (life force) in the body. This is **Hatha Yoga**. The asana is one of several techniques used for controlling the life force in Hatha Yoga. In Raja Yoga words become superfluous; 'I don't think, therefore I am'.

Jana Yoga, the Yoga of Knowledge. It uses the intellect to ask questions, read, reflect and analyse. It transcends the unreal and negates bondage to the material world. It is dependent on words until the mind transcends the intellect.

All paths lead to the union of the individual self with the universal self. You are advised to follow the path that suits your personality but to practise all the other paths to some degree. The usage of words is my own suggestion, to simplify the understanding.

As we hold the postures in a state of bodily concentration and words become superfluous, we may, without realising it, experience this union, if only for a split second. The same applies during the usual final relaxation in a yoga class, and when we meditate.

The Eight Limbs of Raja Yoga
Patanjali compiled and explained the most important elements of yogic theory and practice. 2,000 years ago there were many different schools of yoga and some clarification was necessary. This compilation of yoga sutras represents a climax in thousands of years of yogic development.
It is the practical content of the **Patanjali Sutras** that has received the most recognition. This includes **The Eight Limbs of Raja Yoga**. Some would consider this the 'back bone' of yoga.

Limbs, steps or stages of Raja Yoga

1. Yama, social conduct. **2. Niyama,** personal conduct. **3. Asanas,** postures.
4. Pranayama, control of prana, life force, cosmic energy through breathing. **5. Pratyahara,** withdrawal of the senses.
6. Dharana, concentration. **7. Dhyana,** meditation. **8. Samadhi,** the bliss or super-conscious state.

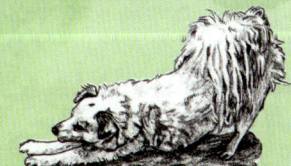

Cautions and Health Issues

People can hurt themselves putting out the garbage, turning over in bed and bending down to pick up something. It is obvious that care must be taken when practising yoga postures. As physical activities go, yoga has a good track record, although one hears of the occasional trapped nerve or accident. Dancers are much more likely to hurt themselves and athletes and football players have a shorter than average life expectancy.

Most of the feedback I have received about my books has been from yoga teachers. A few people told me they practised from them at home and didn't attend a class. These are the ones that need extra guidance and I am writing here with them in mind.

I prefer to distinguish between the fit and unfit, the well-coordinated and the uncoordinated, rather than the beginner and non-beginner. Some people do demanding postures with complete composure and confidence in their first yoga class. Some are used to listening to their bodies: others have lost touch with their bodies and need to develop this skill. Patience is also needed. It is important not to try too hard. Always keep within your comfort zone.

Wait until your body has warmed up before practising demanding stretches and twists.

You are less likely to hurt yourself if you coordinate your breath with your posture work. Always connect to the breath.

Stop if there is any discomfort. Don't hold the postures for too long at first. Move slowly and carefully from one posture to another.

Here are some recognised precautions

If you have a particular physical problem, consult a medical practitioner before starting your practice. Advice varies; if in doubt, seek a second opinion.

If you have **high blood pressure**, it is advisable not to lower your head below the heart, unless you are used to doing this with no ill effects. Care is also needed in inverted postures[1], e.g. the **Head Stand** and **Shoulder Stand.** Taking the hips above the head may not be advisable, although some people with high blood pressure are quite comfortable in inverted postures. Some experimentation is necessary.

Pregnant women should lie on their left-hand side during relaxation. Also, they should not put pressure on the abdomen by lying face downwards.

If you have a **heart problem** or are **pregnant,** don't hold your breath for more than about ten seconds.

Avoid inverted postures if you suffer from **glaucoma, detached retina, neck problems** or have an **ear infection.** Some **pregnant** women are fine doing them: others may faint or have difficulty, so proceed with great caution.

When you are inverted, do not turn your head from side to side. Always look upwards.

Neck and **back problems** vary greatly. Find out which postures help your condition and avoid those that don't. Your medical practitioner should be able to advise you if necessary.

If you have taken **pain killers,** take care not to over-stretch during your posture work as signals to the brain will be suppressed.

If you have had a **hip replacement,** avoid movements like the **Swinging Gate** on page **59** in the **Gate Variations.** Follow the advice of your medical practitioner.

---

1. The only inverted postures in this book are in the **Floor and Wall Sequence** on pages **71** and **72.**

The Full Yogic Breath

I CONSIDER the **Full Yogic Breath** to be one of the most important things I have learnt in my life. Unfortunately I was not taught it until I did my Yoga Teachers Training Course at the age of 52. Meditation comes close behind in order of importance, because good breathing is a prerequisite to good meditation. High upper chest breathing, with lack of harmony between the diaphragm and the abdomen, will limit the development of your meditation.

Method

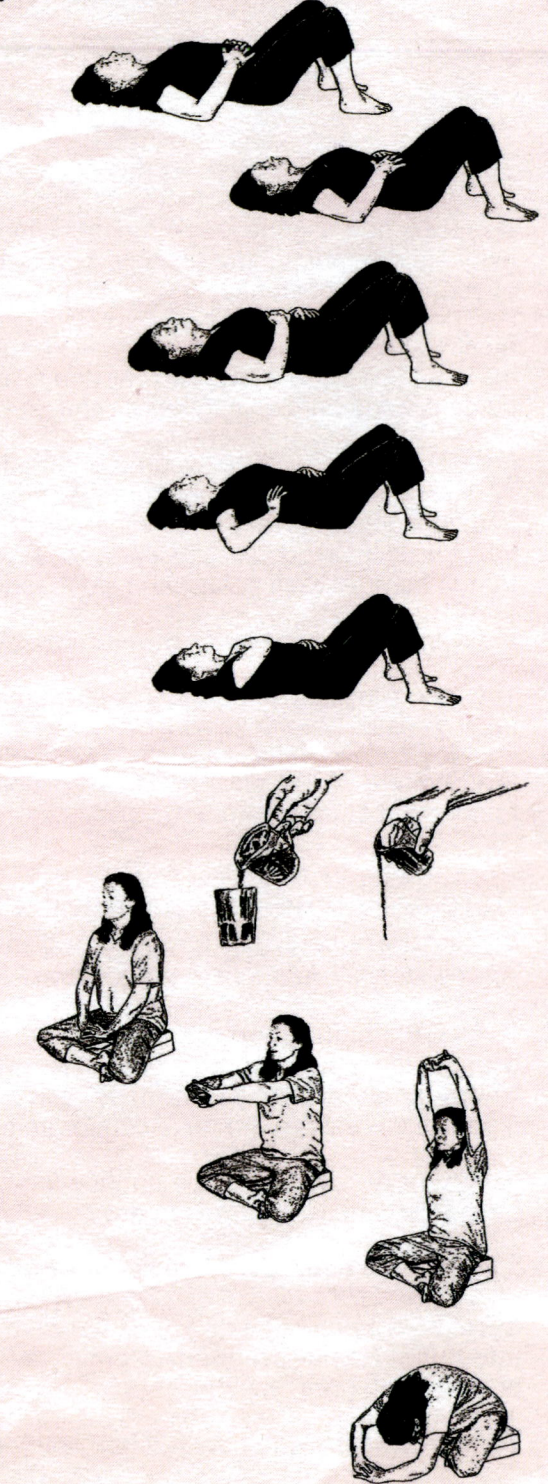

1. Lie on your back. The legs can be straight or slightly bent. Place your hands on the lower abdomen. Breathe with a completely relaxed abdomen. You will feel the abdomen rise on the inhalation, under the influence of the diaphragm, and flatten on the exhalation as the diaphragm contracts up into the rib cage. **Diaphragmatic breathing** brings air into the bottom part of your lungs.

2. Keep the left hand on the abdomen and place your right hand on the diaphragm. Direct your breath to the bottom of your lungs. Feel both hands rising and falling with the breath. *Repeat three times.*

3. Place your right hand half way up the right side of the rib cage. The thumb should be at the back and your fingers wrapped around the front of your ribs. INHALE into the middle part of your lungs. The ribs should move up and out to the sides on the inhalation, and lower on the exhalation. The abdomen will also rise and fall with the breath. *Repeat three times.*

4. Place your right hand on the upper chest and INHALE into the top part of the lungs. The right hand will rise as the sternum, ribs and area below the neck (the clavicles) lift up and out. The left hand on the abdomen will not rise as the diaphragm is passive. *Repeat three times.*

5. Now use all areas of the lungs; bottom, middle and top. This is the **Full Yogic Breath**. As you INHALE, fill the lungs from the bottom upwards, as if you were filling a glass of water. Both hands will rise. EXHALE from the top to the bottom, as if you were emptying a glass of water. Both hands will lower. *Repeat three times.*

6. Sit in **Easy Pose** with the legs lightly crossed, or in another comfortable sitting position. Interlock the fingers in **Venus Loc**k. Lower your hands with the palms facing downwards. EXHALE completely and then INHALE into the bottom part of the lungs. Feel everything around the waist expand.

7. Continue to INHALE as you bring your arms up parallel to the floor, and breathe into the middle part of the lungs. Feel the ribs move up and out.

8. Raise your hands above your head and fill the top part of your lungs. Push away with the palms of your hands. This lifts the rib cage even further. Hold briefly.

9. To EXHALE reverse the procedure. Lower your hands slowly as you empty the lungs from top, middle to bottom. To completely empty the bottom part of the lungs, soften the elbows and lean forward and down. Use the abdominal muscles to squeeze the last bit of air out. INHALE the head up. Repeat from **6** to **9** three times.

Breathing

The breath is very important in yogic thinking. When we inhale, we not only take in oxygen, we take in **prana** (life force or cosmic energy) and breathing is our link to the cosmos. When we inhale, we think of building up a store of energy in the abdomen. It is psychologically healthy to be aware of this grounding, calming and strengthening force in the abdomen.

Traditionally, the yogic inhalation has been with a relaxed abdomen. This is how animals and babies breathe when they are relaxed. When they are active and agitated, the activity can move higher up into the lungs. When you breathe, your whole trunk from the top of your thighs to half way up the neck should move. Scientists have picked up minute movements in the bones of the skull during the breathing process.

As the diaphragm flattens and extends, everything around the waist should move. When I was studying singing at the Guildhall School of Music in the 60s, I was taught to expand around the waist when I breathed in. The abdominal muscles engage automatically on the exhalation to support the outgoing breath. I had the good fortune to come across a copy of **The Week** magazine in my dentist's waiting room. It contained an article about Tanya Streeter who held the record for deep sea diving at that time. She could hold her breath for 6 minutes and 17 seconds. She said that when she got ready to dive, she breathed in so much air that her stomach swelled up until it looked as if she was six months pregnant. We need not go to such extremes!

In Pilates, a slight contraction of the abdomen is recommended on the inhalation. This is understandable as Pilates was created with the ballet dancer in mind. An expanded abdomen would spoil the body line for dancing. Also, the abdominal muscles support the spine during movement. I went to one yoga class where the teacher taught Pilates breathing and decided it was definitely not for me, but yoga can accommodate differences of opinion.

Practising yoga makes you aware of your breathing and the potential expansion of the rib cage. Many people breathe in an unhealthy way for most of their lives. Yoga can correct this. You are never too old to take up yoga. I took my Yoga Teachers Training course at the age of 52. I wasn't particularly flexible. By the time I reached my 60s, I was much more flexible and I had more energy. More importantly, I became a more compassionate, aware human being. Interestingly, the very talented Horoscope writer, the late Jonathan Cainer, wrote just before I took my Yoga TTC, 'You are about to start a new career and it is going to be very good for your social life'. That has proved to be very accurate. Yet another perk that comes with the yoga journey.

Most people breathe between fifteen and twenty times a minute. The breath is closely linked to mental activity. When we are agitated, we breathe quickly. When we listen acutely, we stop breathing. When we slow down our breathing, we become calm.

Experimenting with breath and emotions

To experience this connection, experiment with feeling different emotions. Observe the speed of your breathing and which parts of the body are moving. Here are some suggestions:

Imagine you are relaxing in a hot bath

Feel very angry

You are warm and cosy in bed and about to fall asleep

Feel very frightened

Imagine you are stroking an animal you love very much

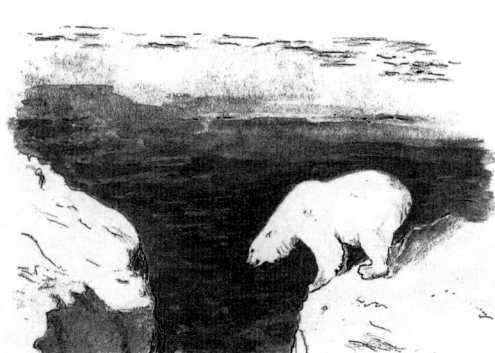

Imagine you are an actor or musician about to perform a demanding part

Feel very happy

Feel very sad

Imagine you are about to meet somebody who is important to you. You haven't seen them for a long time and you are both excited and apprehensive

Extending the Breath

This idea came from Sam Settle, Director of the Prison Phoenix Trust. This charity teaches yoga and meditation to prisoners and gives spiritual guidance. Sam said the simple movements provide a framework through which to lengthen the breath. We do this through counting on the inhalations and exhalations and slowly increasing the counting.

Some yoga teachers insist that the inhalation should be twice as long as the exhalation. This is to prevent hyperventilation. Others find equal inhalations and exhalations quite acceptable. I use both and find that some pupils have a preference for one or the other.

We will start breathing five times a minute. The inhalation and exhalation add up to 12 seconds, with a 4/8 or 6/6 ratio. This is the Coherent Breath of Drs Richard Brown and Patricia Gerbar, see page **13**. It activates the parasympathetic nervous system via the Vagus nerve. I have taught classes where we have breathed five times a minute throughout the class (to a 6/6 or 4/8 ratio) and pupils find this very beneficial.

When you are familiar with the sequence of movements you can start to extend the breath using your chosen ratio.

IN	OUT
6	6
7	7
8	8
10	10
12	12
14	14
15	15

IN	OUT
4	8
5	10
6	12
7	14
8	16
9	18
10	20

When you feel you have reached your comfortable limit, stop increasing the counting. You may find your stamina varies from day to day but your breaths should lengthen with patient practice. On the other hand, if you are a deep sea diver, you may be comfortable with much higher counts, e.g. a four minute breath.

1. Stand with the feet a hip-width apart and your hands by your sides. **INHALE** as you swing your hands above your head. You may choose to lean backwards and look up at your hands.
Count either 4 or 6.

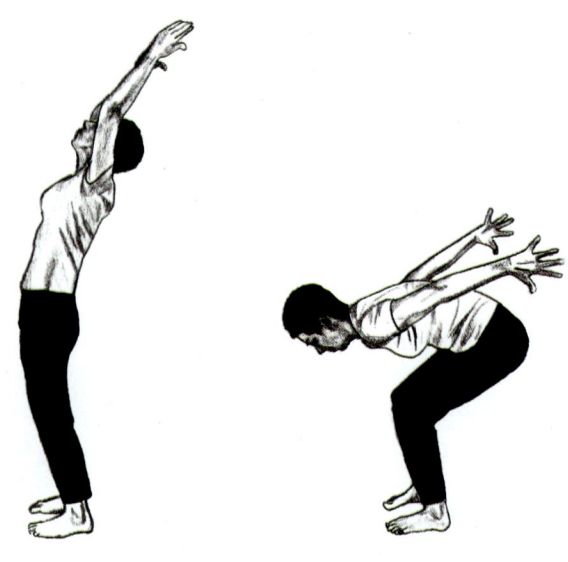

2. **EXHALE** as you sink into a squat and swing your hands back, as illustrated.
Count either 8 or 6.

> You may choose not to bend the knees in 2 and 4.
> If you have high blood pressure, do not lower the head below the heart.

3. Proceed as in **1**, but when you INHALE, rise up on your toes.
Keep counting in your chosen ratios.

4. EXHALE back into the squat. You can either stay on tip-toes or lower the heels to the floor.

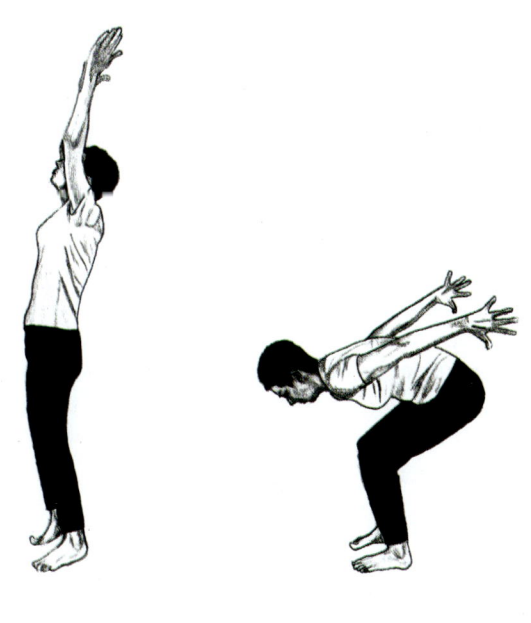

The HA Breath

This involves **inhaling** through the nose and **exhaling** through the mouth.

It can be **voiced**, with a loud **Ha**, but it is usually **unvoiced**, i.e. whispered and similar to **Ujjayi** breathing.

The vowel sound does not have to be an **Ah**. It can be a neutral sound like **Er**. The **H** consonant at the beginning gives it definition.

---

5. From the squat, INHALE the hands up as before with the heels on the floor.

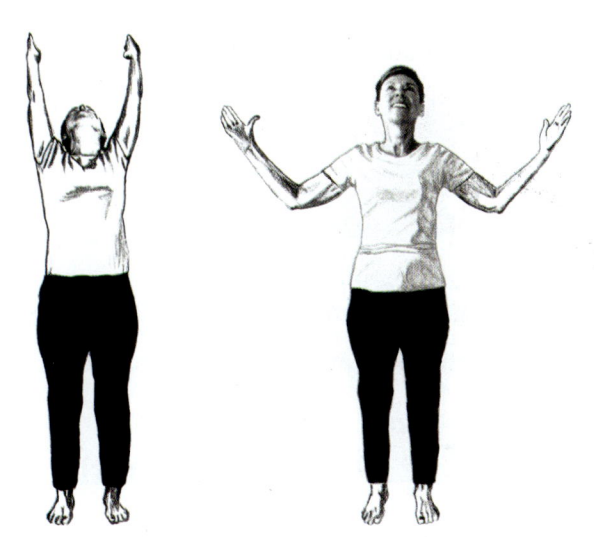

6. EXHALE as you swing your hands out to the sides into **Open Heart** pose. Move your shoulders back and down. Breathe out through your mouth with a **HA Breath** (see box).

7. INHALE as you bend the knees and swing the arms round in front, as illustrated.

8. EXHALE as you straighten the knees, lower the arms to your sides and stretch up to your full height. Tuck in the tail-bone. Lower the chin a little and stretch the back of your neck.
Enjoy the feeling of stretching to your full height. Be aware of the sensations in your feet. You are likely to lift the inner arches.

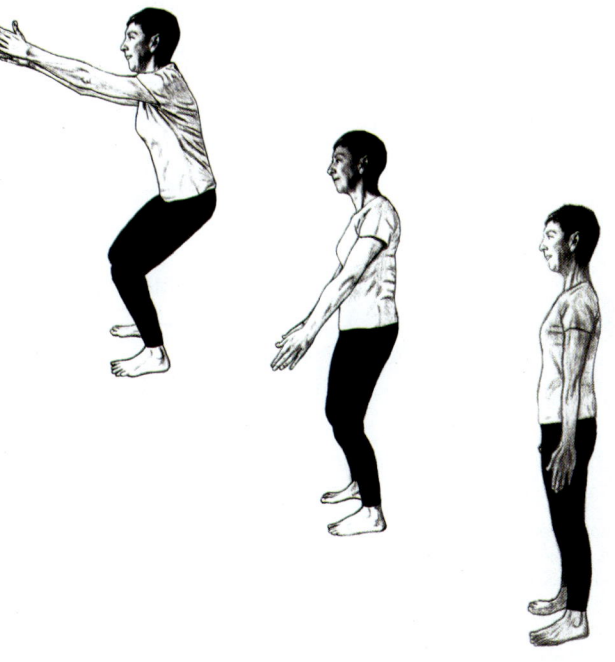

Repeat about three times and when you feel ready, continue, using one of the other suggested breathing combinations.

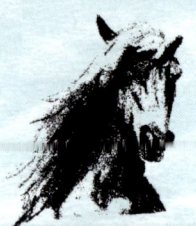

The Sympathetic and Parasympathetic Nervous Systems

THE NETWORK of nerves that connect to the spinal cord and brain (the Peripheral Nervous System) has two overlapping parts. They are the somatic (under conscious control) and autonomic (self-regulating).

The **Autonomic Nervous System** normally functions outside conscious, willed control[1]; e.g. regulating breathing, digestion and pupil dilation. It has two counteracting parts, the **Sympathetic** and **Parasympathetic**.

Sympathetic

Bodily functions speed up.

There is a high consumption of energy with some wastage of energy.

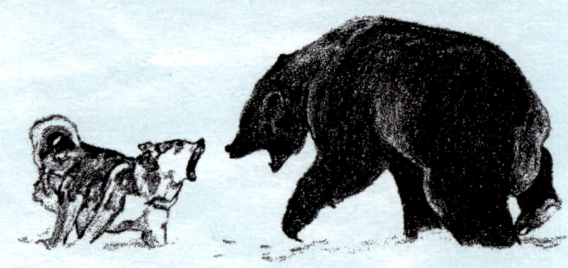

It operates when we are in **Survival Mode**[2]. This is the **Fight or Flight** response. In a frightening, life-threatening situation we have to react quickly by either attacking the threat or running away. This can be a sudden, dramatic happening or a continual sense of unease[3].

The system speeds up the heartbeat, sends more blood to the relevant muscles and enlarges the pupils of the eye to enable it to use all available light. It takes blood away from the digestive tract and sends it to the parts that need to react to the emergency. Feeding and reproduction can be part of the survival mode.

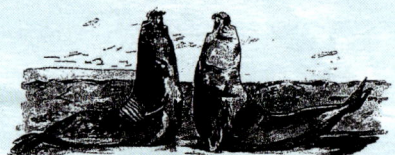

Body Language

Movements speed up. There is an emphasis of movement in the hands, nose and face. In extreme cases there will be quick upper chest **Nose Breathing**.

The obvious example is the backward ears and flared nostrils of a horse when it is angry, frightened or threatened. One of my pupils says her husband flares his nostrils when he is angry.

This newspaper headline describes a woman defending herself in debate. ***Nostrils flaring, face flushed, she snapped: He's just wrong***[4].

Parasympathetic

Bodily functions slow down.

There is a low consumption of energy with some storage of energy.

It operates when we are secure, confident and contented.

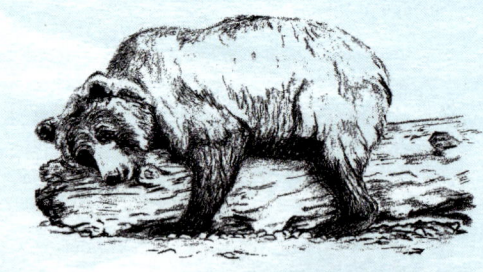

The **Four Rs** are usually used to describe its activities:
Rest, Relax, Restore and **Renew**.

The heart slows down and the digestive system is well supplied with blood. The pupils contract as orientation turns inwards, away from external things.

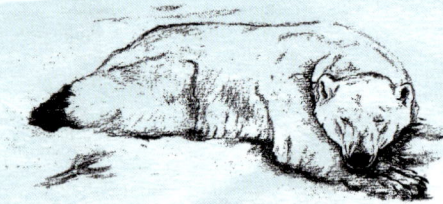

Body Language

Movements slow down.

The hands and face become passive.

Breathing is lower down in the body. There is more diaphragm awareness and abdominal movement.

When humans and animals are deeply relaxed, **Throat Breathing (Ujjayi)** occurs naturally. It is not unusual to hear a human or dog breathing through a slightly closed throat while sleeping or dozing.

1. *It is possible to control the heart beat and other bodily functions but it takes practise and concentration. Some yogis and military personnel, for example, have trained themselves to do this (see The Psychic Warrior, by David Morehouse, ISBN 978-190-2636207).*
2. *All creatures with a backbone, e.g. humans, animals and fish, have this basic mechanism.*
3. *Swami Ambikananda, from Reading, UK, said in a workshop that she had asked a cancer specialist why so many people had cancer today. He said, Because there is too much use of the Sympathetic Nervous System.*
4. *The Daily Mail, 30.1.08.*

Preparatory information relating to the next two sequences.
They combine movements with the breath to relieve anxiety, depression, traumatic stress and most psychological problems that affect our well-being.

These quotations are from videos on the **Breath Body Mind** website. The doctors are in discussion with students.

1. **Dr Gerbarg** is explaining why the breath is so powerful.

Of all the autonomic functions of the body, breathing is the only one that we can voluntarily control. You can't easily, voluntarily change your heart beat or digestion, but you can change your pattern of breathing any time you wish. So breathing gives us a portal of entry where we can directly access and send messages to the interceptive system.

If we can figure out the language, if we can find out the code, and determine which breathing practice is going to send the messages we want to send to the higher control centres to activate them and get them to function better, then we have a chance to, very simply, change the way our emotions are regulated.

That's what we find over and over again when we do these studies. If you change the way people are breathing, their emotions change, their anxiety goes down, they become less depressed. We have in our hands a completely self-empowering treatment for the self-regulation of our emotions.

Why is breathing so powerful to the brain? Breathing is essential for our survival. If you don't get any food for a day you are still going to be alive, but if you don't breathe for 3 or 4 minutes you will die. So which messages are going to be received and paid attention to and to be given top priority? Messages from the lungs are going to override any other messages. If you can't breathe, if your airways are obstructed, your entire brain and mental apparatus has to quickly shift and figure out how to keep your airways open.

That's why we believe these practices can work so quickly - literally within minutes.

2. **Dr. Brown** is explaining how breath work harmonises mind, body and spirit.

Normally every function in your mind, body, spirit complex has a diurnal rhythm. There is an hour in the day when you do algebra and differential equations best. There's an hour or two when you are strongest physically. Every function in your mind, body, spirit has its rhythm. The thing is, these rhythms are totally chaotic and incoherent. Your energy is really incoherent.

When you start doing this breathing it's remarkable. You can measure how they all come together. They all align. Instead of your system being like different sections of an orchestra warming up, it becomes like an orchestra playing together and making beautiful music. Your blood-flow and your brain and your heart synchronise. So how often do your head and your heart come together? Not often, but life is much better when they do.

For further information go to www.Breath-Body-Mind.com
They are the authors of The Healing Power of the Breath (2012). Published by Shambhala

The Coherent Breath
The Coherent Breath is defined as slow gentle breathing through the nose at a rate of **5 breaths per minute**. It involves **inhaling** for **6** seconds and **exhaling** for **6** seconds. Dr Brown says this breathing ratio activates the **Vagus Nerve**. This is the nerve associated with the **Parasympathetic Nervous System**. The benefits of this system can be found on the opposite page.

1. **QiGong Breath** for Calmness, Energy and Strength.

Breathing Pattern, in counts roughly a second long:

INHALE for 4 – HOLD for 4 – EXHALE for 6 – HOLD for 2

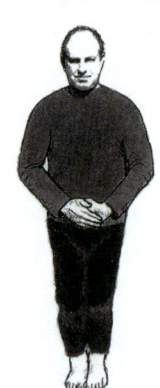 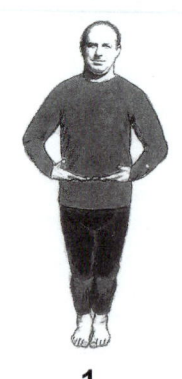 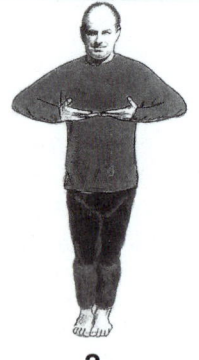 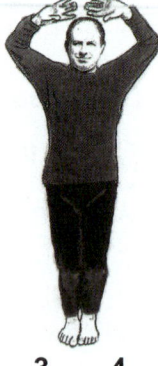

A. Stand with the feet together and the knees soft and slightly bent. Place your hands on the lower abdomen with your dominant hand on top.

B. **INHALE** for **4** counts, starting with your palms facing upwards and bringing them above your head. It will be necessary to rotate the palms away from your body at shoulder level.

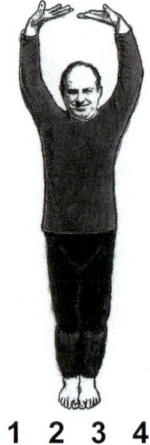 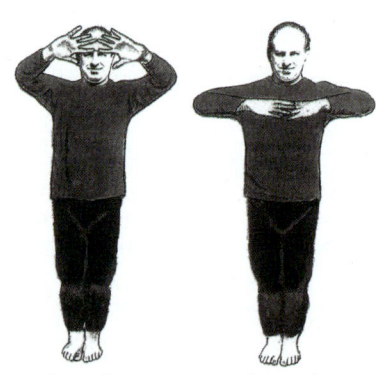 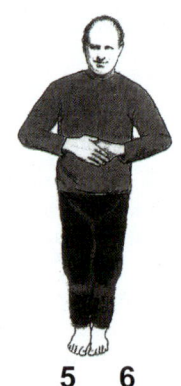

C. **HOLD** for **4** counts with the hands higher above the head, and the elbows straight.

D. **EXHALE** to the count of **6** as you bring your fingers together above your head and lower them till they are hovering just above the waist. At shoulder level your hands will rotate towards the body and your dominant hand will slide on top of the other hand.

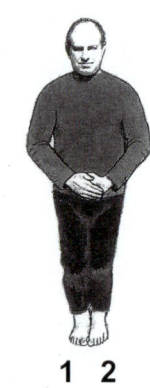 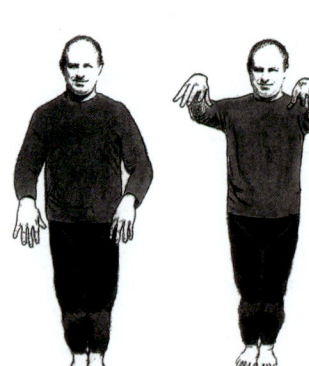 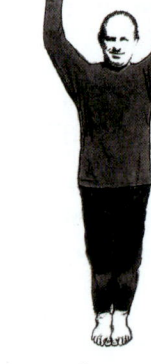

E. HOLD[1] with your hands in the starting position (**A**) for **2** counts.

F. Separate your hands and, with the palms facing downwards and the arms straight, **INHALE** them above your head to the count of **4**. The hands should feel soft and heavy. The fingers will curve downwards naturally. By the fourth count your hands will be above your head with the palms facing.

1. **Caution.**
If you suffer from Chronic Obstructive Pulmonary Disease (COPD) or Emphysema, you may not want to pause for **2** counts after your exhalation in **E** and **I**. You may prefer to **EXHALE** for the count of **8**. I teach it this way in a class.

G. Open the arms out wide and **HOLD** for **4** counts.

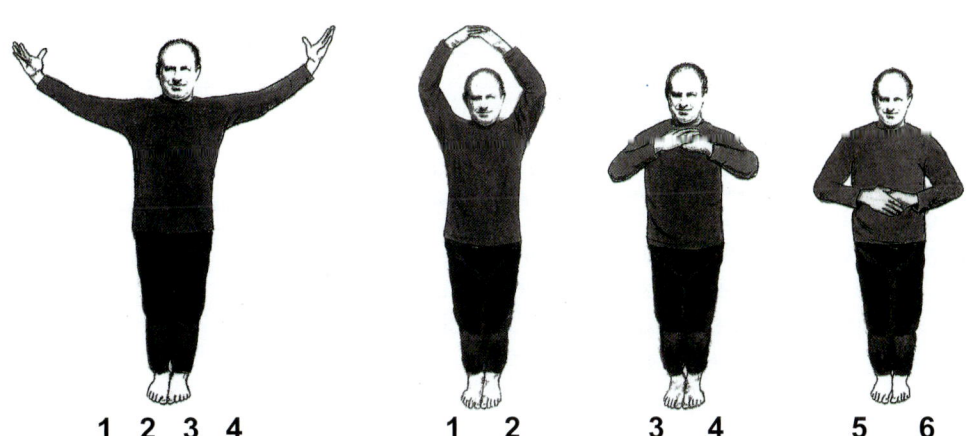

1 2 3 4   1   2   3   4   5   6

H. EXHALE to the count of **6** as you bring the fingers together above your head and lower the hands down, as in **D**. The dominant hand will slide on top of the other hand again.

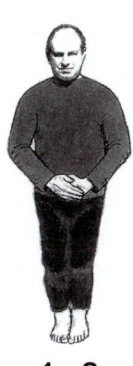

I. Return to **A** and **HOLD** for **2** counts.
Return to B and repeat.

Repeat entire sequence from B, 16 times.
This takes about 5 to 7 minutes.

1 2

Breath ~ Body ~ Mind ©

Practices to relieve stress, anxiety, trauma and depression

I was introduced to these powerful practices at a conference in London organised by Heather Mason of the *Minded Institute* in March, 2015. The title was *Yoga, Key to Mental Health*.

Husband and wife team, Dr Richard P. Brown MD and Dr Patricia L. Gerbarg MD, use these techniques to help victims of disasters around the world. These include the 9/11 World Trade Center attacks, the Haiti earthquake, the Horizon Gulf oil spill, slavery in the Sudan and military service trauma.

Their benefits have been demonstrated in health care practitioners, individuals with psychiatric and medical conditions, research studies and those with the disorders of Post Traumatic Stress (PTSD), Attention Deficit Hyperactivity (ADHD), mood and life stress.

> *The practices improve physical and emotional well-being and are gentle and soft and safe for most people. However, if you experience any physical discomfort, stop and relax. If the discomfort persists, seek the advice of a medical practitioner before continuing. You will need to practise these techniques every day if possible to gain maximum benefits.*

Dr Richard P. Brown MD is Associate Clinical Professor in Psychiatry at Columbia University, NY. He is an Integrative Psychiatrist, Clinical researcher, Mind-Body Qigong, Yoga and Martial Arts teacher. He developed *Breath-Body-Mind* to quickly relieve stress and trauma.

Dr Patricia L Gerbarg MD is a Harvard-trained Psychiatrist, Clinical Researcher, writer, consultant and teaches Neuroscience, integration of *Breath-Body-Mind* with Psychotherapy and natural treatments for mental health.

2. The Great Harmoniser of Breath.

Breathing Pattern
INHALE for **6** – **EXHALE** for **6**.
This is the **Coherent Breath,** see page **12**.

A. Start with the feet apart and the hands on the abdomen. **INHALE** to the count of **6** as you raise your hands above your head. The palms rotate outwards at chest level and then push upwards.

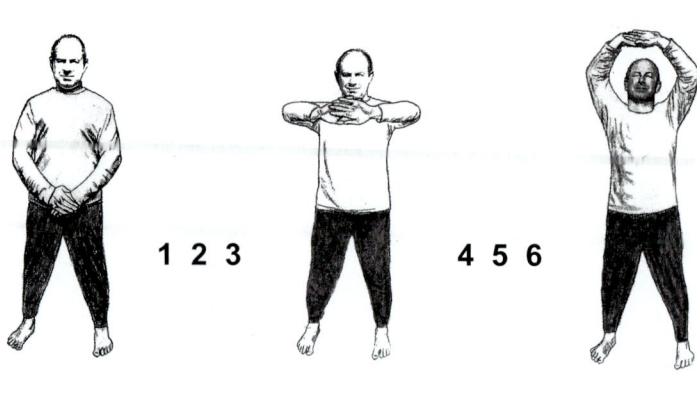

1 2 3   4 5 6

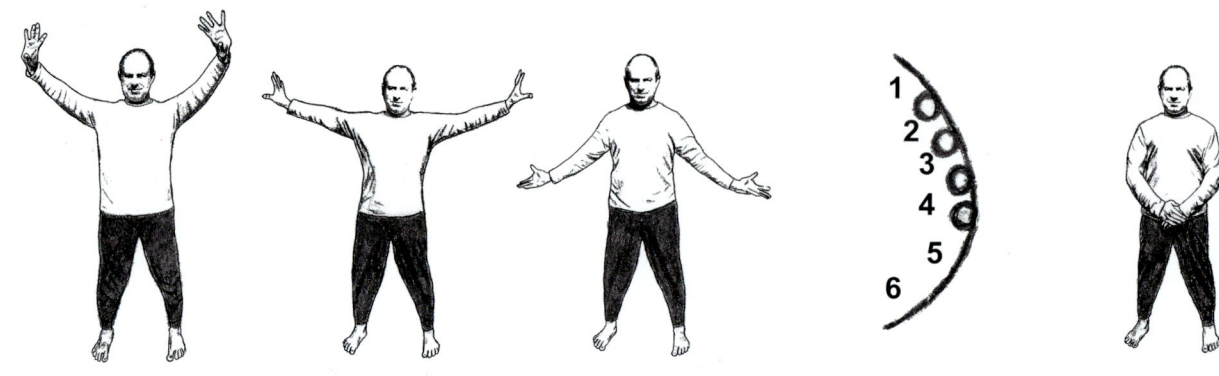

B. Separate the hands and prepare to lower them to the sides in a wide circle. As you **EXHALE** them down to the count of **6**, rotate your wrists **4** times and return your hands to the abdomen (see diagram above).

C. Repeat **A**. **INHALE** as you return your hands above your head.

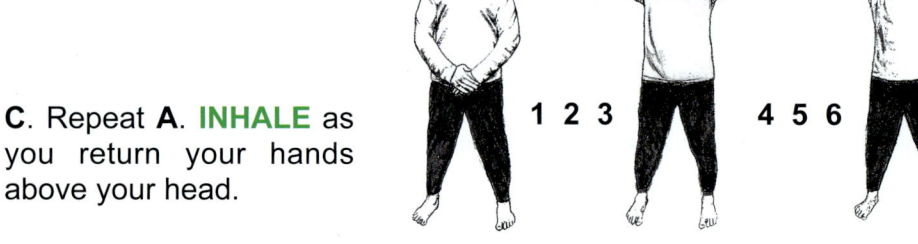

1 2 3   4 5 6

D. **EXHALE** as you circle the hands back down to the starting point with the palms facing downwards. This time, don't rotate the wrists. It is a smooth, flowing movement.

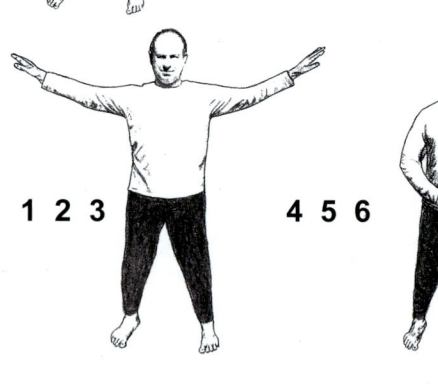

1 2 3   4 5 6

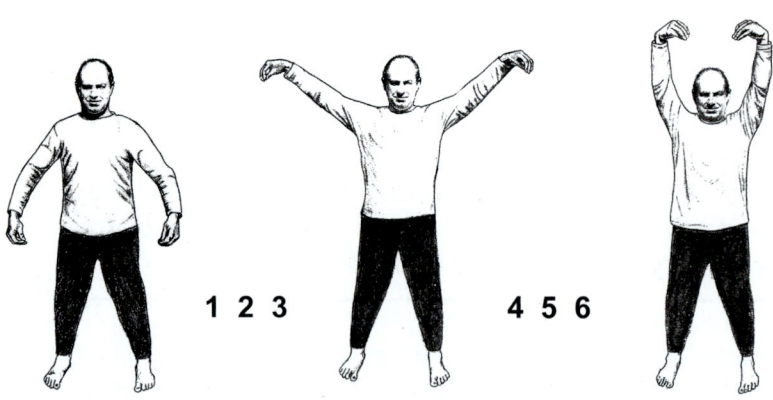

1 2 3   4 5 6

E. Bring your fingers and thumbs together, forming a **Crane Beak** with your hands. **INHALE** them up in a circle. The fingers turn to face each other above your head.

F. As you **EXHALE**, bend forwards from the hips with a flat back, bringing the hands down in front of you. Swing your hands behind you and look forwards. As you count 5 and 6, bring your feet together and bend your knees.

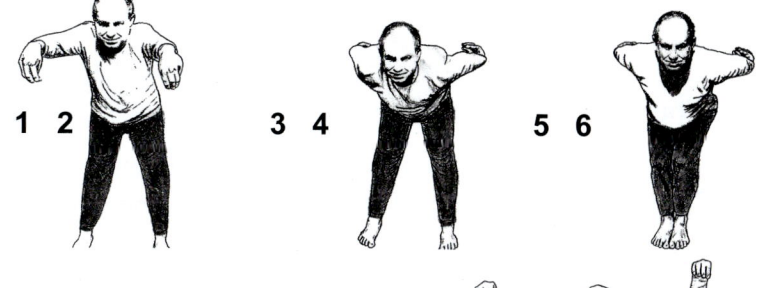

1 2   3 4   5 6

G. **INHALE** as you swing your hands forwards and sink down into a comfortable squat. Feel your weight on the heels. Gradually straighten the legs and bring the hands above your head.

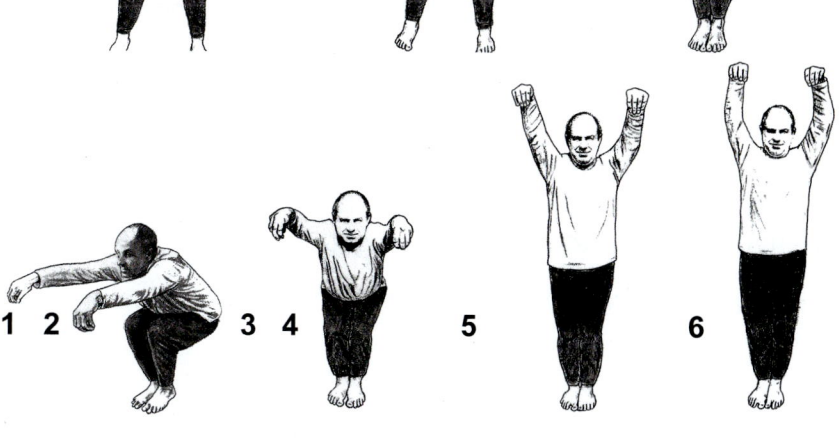

1 2   3 4   5   6

H. EXHALE as you separate your fingers and curve your hands next to your head. Stretch them forwards with the fingers overlapping[1].

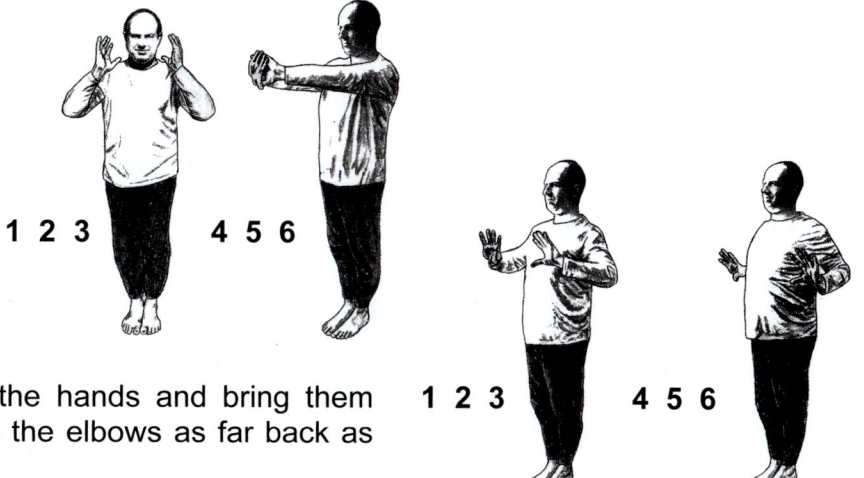

1 2 3   4 5 6

1 2 3   4 5 6

I. INHALE as you separate the hands and bring them back at shoulder height. Take the elbows as far back as you can.

J. EXHALE as you push your palms forwards. As you count **4**, **5** and **6**, step your feet apart and bring your hands back to the lower abdomen, returning to the starting point.

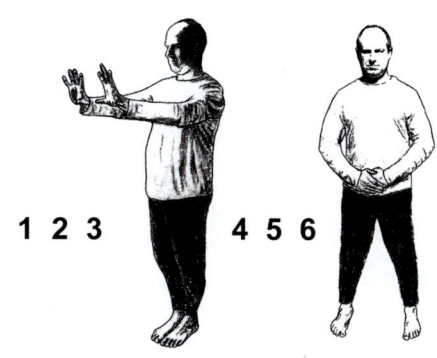

1 2 3   4 5 6

Observations: The same comments and cautions apply to both of these sequences. Both require regular practise. They are more difficult to memorise than you would expect and require deep concentration. This is therapeutic as it stops your mind from wandering off down leafy lanes. This level of concentration, combined with movement and the breath, creates a very powerful practice. This has been the experience of my pupils.

Daily practise of these two sequences should help to relieve anxiety, depression, traumatic stress and most psychological problems that affect our well-being.

1. The movements from **H** to **J** should feel like waves coming and going on the seashore. They can flow smoothly and gracefully like water.

One Side Active, One Side Passive

This is another idea volunteered by Sam Settle, Director of the Prison Phoenix Trust. Sam said the original idea came from Derek Thorne.

It involves making a series of movements with one side of the body while the other side remains uninvolved, soft and relaxed. After doing one side, the difference in feeling in the two sides of the body is often very noticeable.

1. Lie on your back with the palms facing downwards. Elongate the back of your neck and tuck in the chin a little. To make yourself more comfortable, try lifting the hips a little and then plonking them down. Repeat this with your shoulders.

Bring your awareness to the breath and allow yourself to sink heavily into the floor.

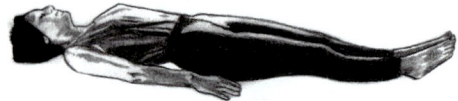

2. INHALE the right leg up. **EXHALE** it down. **x3**

Keep checking the left side of the body to make sure it is not involved with the movements.

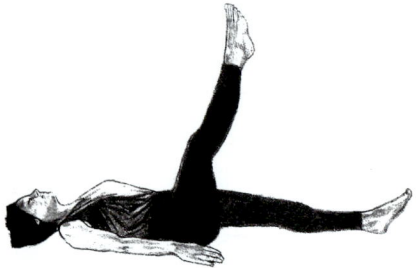

3. INHALE the leg up again and then **EXHALE** as you lower it half way down. Pulse it up and half way down with the breath. **x3**

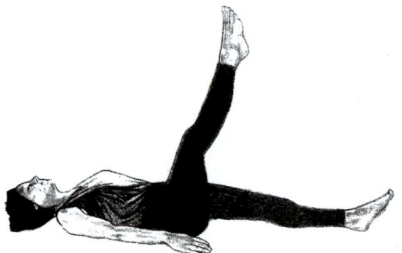
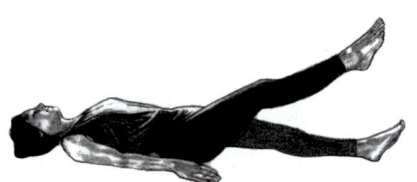

4. INHALE the right knee back towards your head. **EXHALE** as you straighten it and lower it down. **x3** Keep checking your left side. Keep it soft and relaxed. **INHALE** it back, without the foot touching the floor

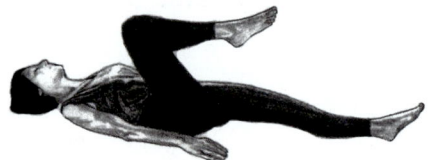
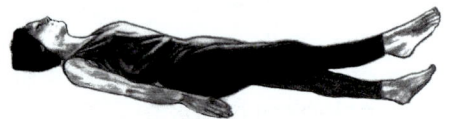

5. Bring your right knee back and guide it in circles with your right hand. Start with small circles and then move to larger circles. Change direction and reverse, starting with larger circles and then making smaller ones.

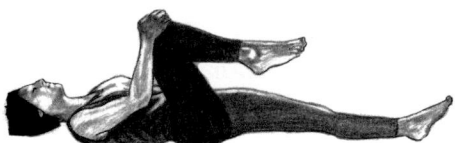

6. INHALE as you pull the right knee down and back to the side firmly with your hand. **EXHALE** as you remove your hand and stretch your right arm back and your foot forwards and down, pointing the toes. The hand and foot don't touch the floor. Hold for at least three breaths as you stretch along your right side. **x3**

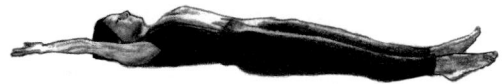

7. Catch hold of your right foot with your right hand and straighten the leg up towards the ceiling. Pull the leg back. You may need to keep the knee bent a little.

If you find this difficult, you can place your hand on the calf or thigh. Encourage the leg back towards the head. Hold for about 8 breaths.

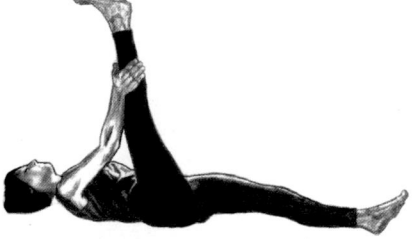

8. When you are ready, return your hand to the floor and begin to lower the leg very slowly, breathing normally, taking about 20 seconds, until the foot is about 6 inches above the floor. Hold it there for as long as you comfortably can.

While you are lowering and holding the leg about 6 inches above the floor, pay particular attention to the sensations on the different sides of the body.

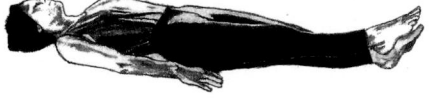

9. Carefully lower your leg to the floor. Observe the difference in the sensations between your right and left sides. The right side is likely to feel longer than the left. It may feel lighter and as if it has lost its form.

With your eyes closed, you may feel that you know which way your feet are pointing, but when you look, the angle is different. You may want to discuss this between yourselves. A few people don't feel any difference so don't worry if you are one of them.

When you are ready, change sides and repeat.

Circling Warm Up

This sequence involves making circling movements. Your body should remain relaxed and soft throughout. Let it flow like a river in a continuous, free-flowing movement.

While making circles, you will find yourself inhaling at a certain point, usually when the trunk of your body expands, and exhaling when it contracts. Try to make the exhalations longer than the inhalations. The speed of your rotations will be regulated by your breath capacity. Try to breathe slowly.

It is necessary to count the rotations so that you make the same number in each direction. You could make between 5 and 10 rotations in each direction and you may feel you want to vary the numbers in different postures. A certain amount of experimentation is necessary and you are likely to develop your own system of breathing and counting.

Sources

Most of the ideas come from general yoga repertoire. **5** and **6** are inspired by ideas from US-based Micheline Berry's DVDs. The idea for **11** comes from a Kundalini Yoga book, **Tree Yoga**, by Satya Singh and Fred Hagender[1]. They suggest that you keep your eyes closed and focus on the point between the eyebrows (the Third Eye). This adds a different dimension to the movements. You may choose to follow this suggestion while circling in some of the other postures.

1. Lie on your back with the knees bent and the feet crossed. The hands rest on the knees. With the knees touching, rotate them in small clockwise circles.
After at least 5 rotations, allow the knees to move further apart. Start to make middle-sized circles.
After the same number of rotations, start to make the circles as large as you can with the knees wide apart.

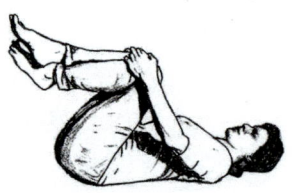

Pause briefly and then change the direction of the circles but start with large circles and proceed in reverse order. You will pass through middle-sized circles and finish up with small anti-clockwise circles and the knees together.

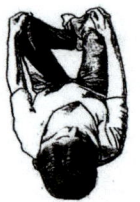
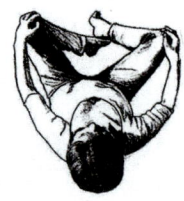

2. Lie on your back with your hands by your sides and the palms facing downwards. Bend your knees with the feet at least a hip-width apart. Push up on your heels with your toes pointing upwards and lift your hips a few inches off the floor.
Circle the hips in a clockwise direction, up to the left and then as high as you can. Lower down to the right and pass through the starting point without the hips touching the floor.

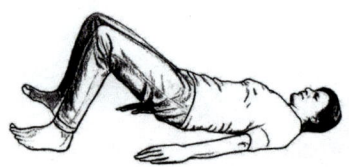

After completing your chosen number of circles, pause briefly, and *repeat in the opposite direction*.

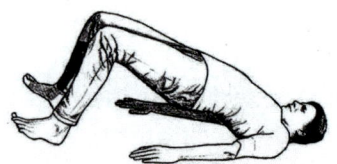

3. Shoulder Circling. Sit in **Easy Pose** with the legs crossed or in any comfortable position. Place your hands on your knees. Lean forwards with the elbows bent. When you circle backwards your elbows will be straight and your chin tucked in. Continue round to the left. *Change direction* after your chosen number of circles.

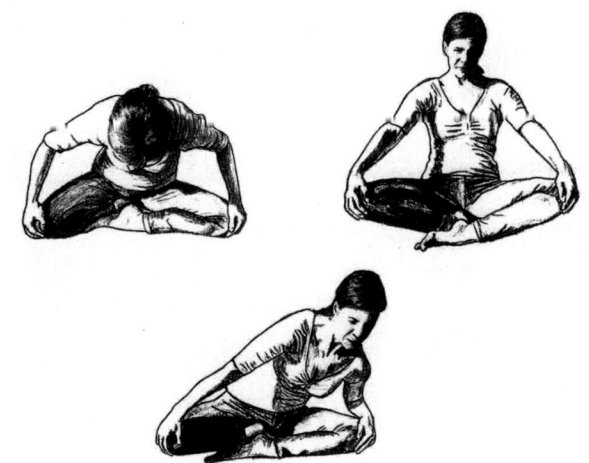

4. Rib Cage Circling. From the same starting position, feel as if the top of your head is being pulled upwards. Circle the rib cage clockwise. The head will make smaller circles than in **3**. *Change direction* when you are ready.

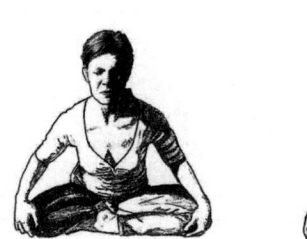
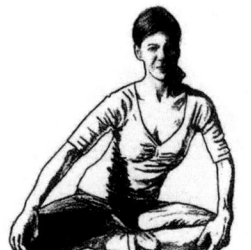

5. Sit with your knees bent and the feet about 9 inches apart. Clasp your hands with the palms together and the fingers wrapped round the sides of your hands.
Make large circles with the hands. When you circle forwards stretch as far forwards as you can. When you are in the backward position, pause briefly with the hands resting on the chest. *Change direction* when you are ready.

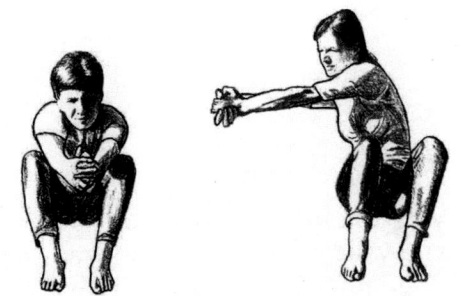

6. From the same starting position, separate your hands and stretch them forwards with the palms facing but not touching.
As you circle round, follow your hands around with your eyes. When you are leaning backwards, they will be high above your head and when you are forwards they will be low. *Change direction* when you are ready.

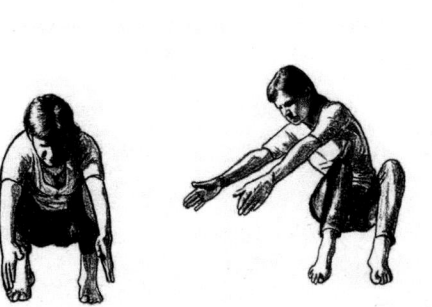
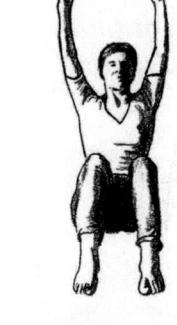
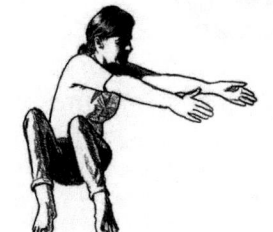

7. Circling Cat. This involves circling up and down in the **Cat** posture. Start in an 'all fours' position with the knees slightly apart and the hands under the shoulders. You may choose to turn the fingers inwards.

Bend the elbows, lowering the chin a short distance from the floor. Circle up to the left and push up as high as you can before lowering to the right. Continue for your chosen number of circles.
Change direction and repeat.

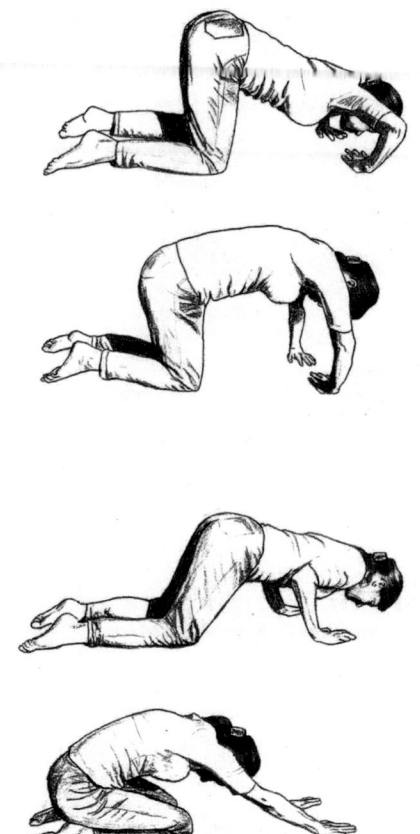

8. This involves circling forwards and backwards in the **Circling Cat**. Start with the hands facing forwards. Swing forwards over your hands. Circle to the right and then as far back as you can so that the hips touch the heels and your arms are straight. Complete your circle to the left and ***continue until you are ready to change direction.***

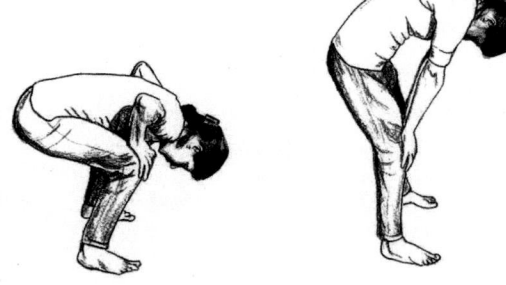

9. Circling in the Standing Cat. Stand with the feet a hip-width apart. Bend your knees and place your hands on them. Lower down into a deep squat and then circle up to the left. Push up into a **Standing Downward Cat** before lowering to the right.
Continue until you are ready to change direction.

10. Hip Circling. Stand with the feet a hip-width apart. Place your hands on your hips. Make large clockwise circles with your hips.
Change direction and repeat.

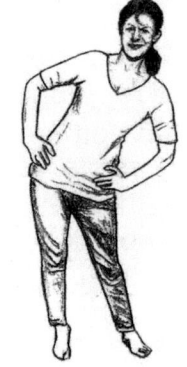
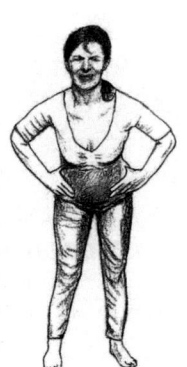

11. Stand with the feet a hip-width apart. Join your hands together above your head. Clasp the fingers together with the first fingers stretched out and the thumbs crossed over[2]. Make large circles with your arms and upper body. When your hands are forwards, your hips will move backwards and vice versa. Flow like a river. ***Change direction and repeat.***

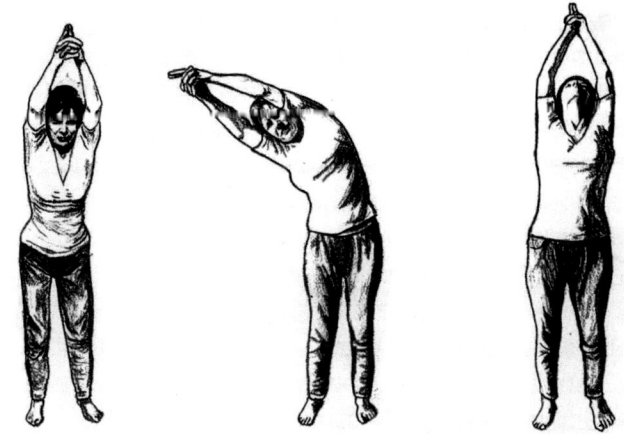

12. Churning the Mill. Sit with your legs wide apart and your toes towards your head. Push away with your heels. Join your hands together in **Venus Lock** with the palms facing outwards. Make your chosen number of large circles with your hands in both directions.

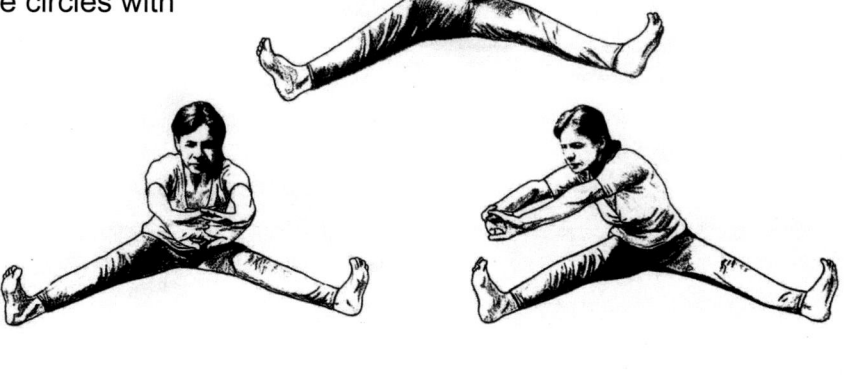

13. Churning the Mill in Pairs. If possible, pair up with somebody whose legs are the same length as yours.

Sit opposite each other with the soles of the feet together. Clasp your hands in **Fireman's Lock**, catching hold of each other's wrists.

Continue as in **12**. When one of you is pulling the other one forward, you may like to pause briefly to experience the benefit of the posture (the decompression of the spine). ***Change sides and repeat.***

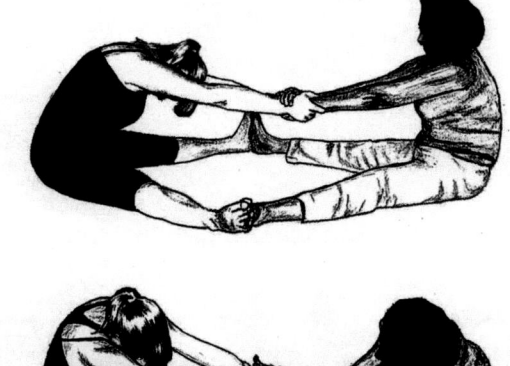

1. Tree Yoga, published by Findhorn Press (2006) ISBN 978-1-84409-119-5
2. See Ksepana Mudra, page 49

Native American Planting Chant

I was introduced to this chant at a North Hampshire BWY day in Aldershot in 2011 and subsequently taught my own version of it in my classes. I found a seated version was very much enjoyed in old people's homes. It has obvious appeal to children and serves as light relief in adult classes. It can also serve as a prelude to more demanding postures as it warms the body.

I have tried to get as close as possible to the original version but this has proved difficult. The teacher in Aldershot said she was taught the chant by Simon Heather who is a frequent attraction at Yoga Festivals and events with his chanting workshops[1]. I contacted Simon who directed me to the CD, *Turn the World Around, 28 Chants and Community Songs,* by Eagle's Wing, Centre of Contemporary Shamanism. It is called *Ploughing Chant* in their booklet. Mutations and variations are inevitable in communal art forms that are not documented at their source. The melody is taken from the CD but I cannot verify the authenticity of the movements. They have probably evolved from many sources.

I am presenting two different versions. The first is the one I was taught at the BWY day with the addition of **6** and **7** which are my suggestions. The second version involves the incorporation of information I received from Simon Heather. I now combine both versions in my classes.

Here is the melody for **HEY YA NA NA**

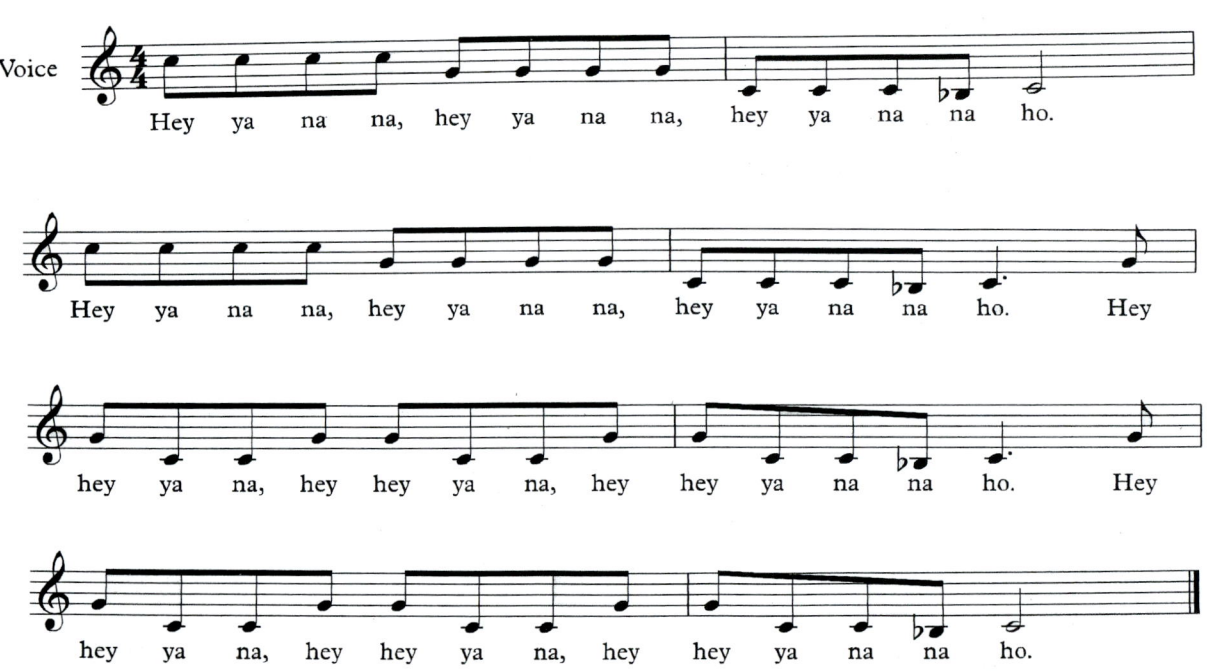

Version 1

When movements are repeated, the size of the drawings is reduced.

> **Please note.** Each line of the music is repeated. Do each set of movements and the chorus twice.

1. **Planting the Seeds**. Dance/step round in a circle.

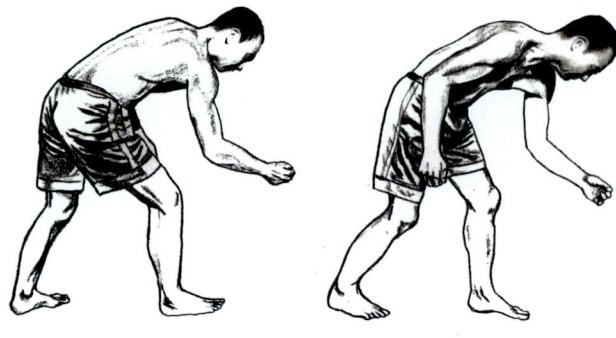

HEY YA NA NA,   **HEY YA NA NA,**

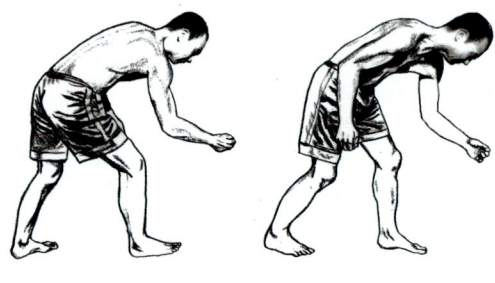

HEY YA NA NA,   **HO**   **x2**

2. This is the Chorus which is repeated after every new idea.

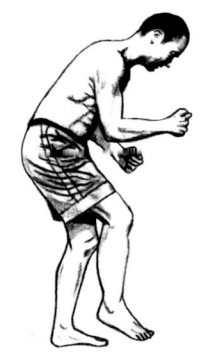 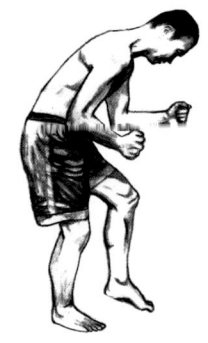 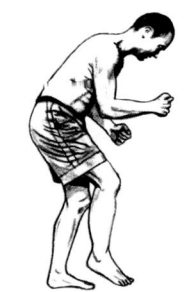 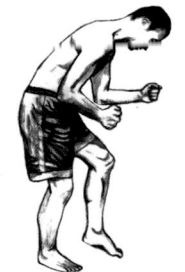

HEY HEY YA NA,　　　**HEY HEY YA NA,**　　　**HEY HEY YA NA NA**　　　**HO**　　**x2**

3. The Rain Falls.

Lower both hands, imitating the rain falling down by fluttering the fingers.

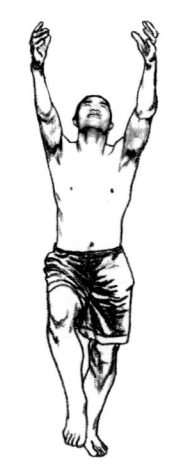 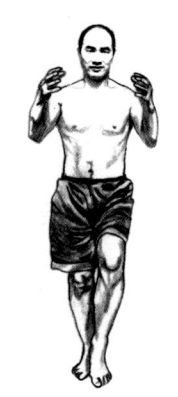 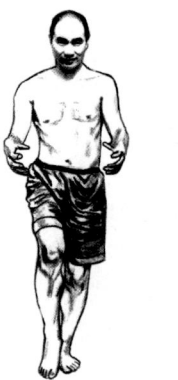 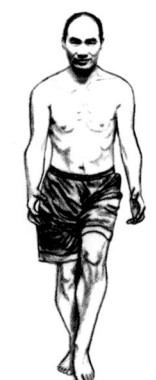

HEY YA NA NA,　　**HEY YA NA NA,**　　**HEY YA NA NA,**　　**HO**

4. The Wind Blows.

Sway your hands from side to side above your head.

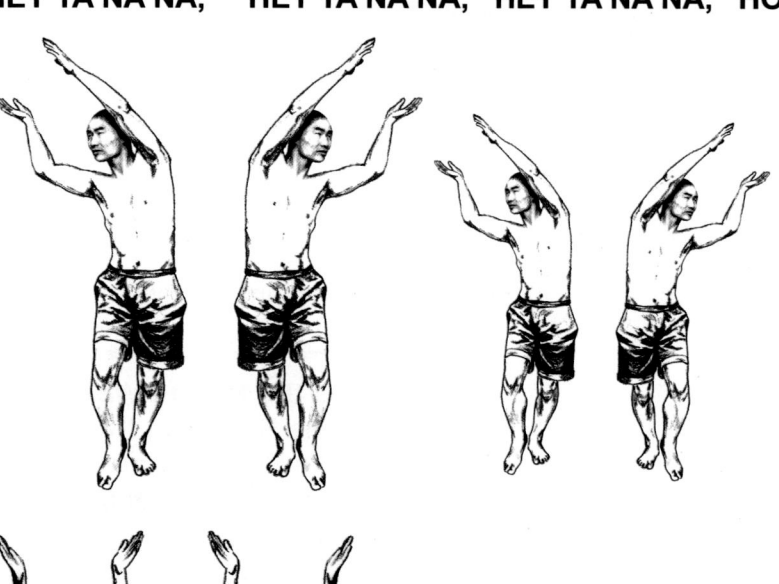

5. The Sun Shines.

Imitate the sun's rays with the hands above your head.

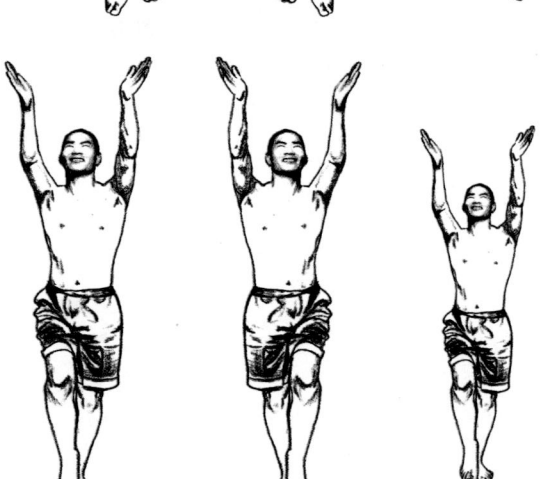 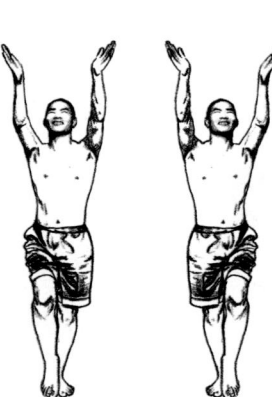

6. Picking the Crops. Lean forward and stretch out to pick the crops[2].

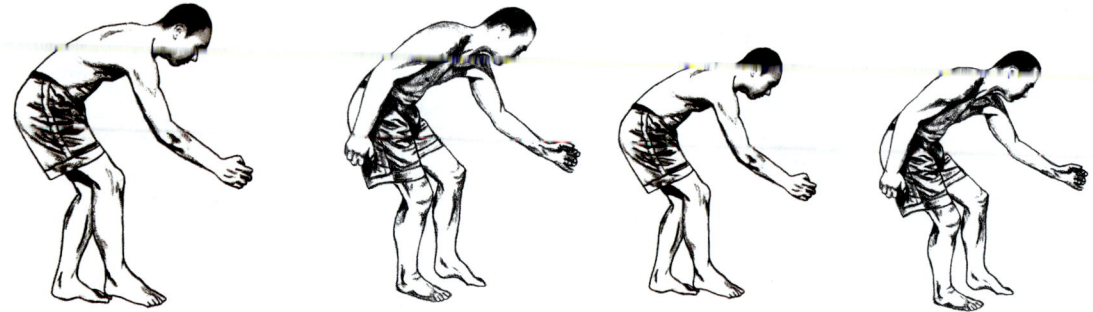

7. Picking the Fruit from the Trees. Stretch up and pick the fruit.

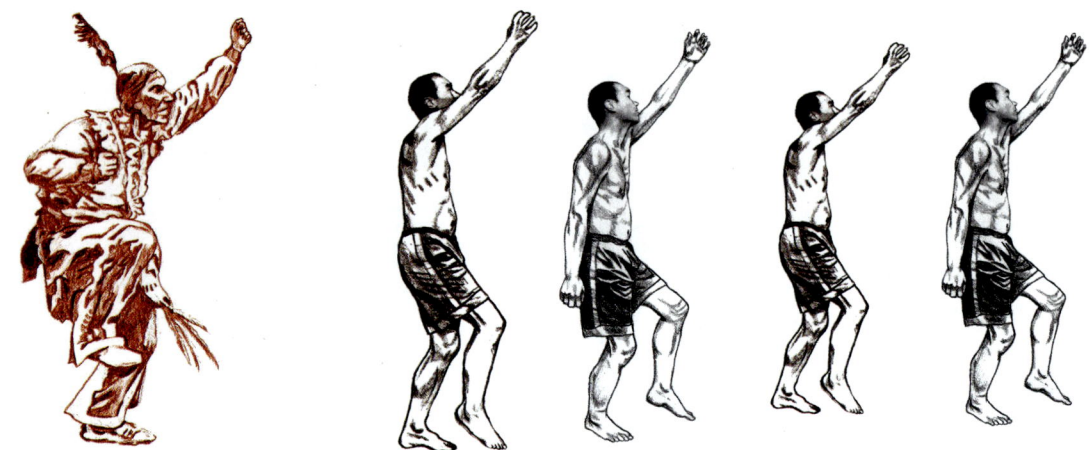

This is taken from a sketch of a Ghost Dance of the Lakota tribe of North and South Dakota, c.1800.

To Conclude – Slow down the **Chorus** and sing it loudly and purposefully.

Version 2

The **Planting Song** celebrates the four elements[3] with different hand movements as you move round in a circle.

> **Stamping the Feet to Wake Up the Earth**
> **Sowing the Seeds on the Earth (Air)**
> **Calling the Rain to Water the Seeds**
> **Calling the Sun to Ripen the Corn**
> **Thanking Great Spirit**

This version requires a different mindset. We are not just imitating the subject matter, we are invoking the elements and then giving thanks.

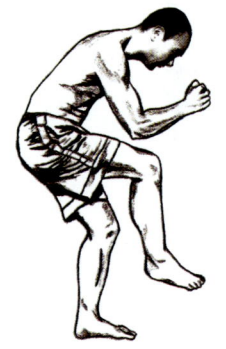
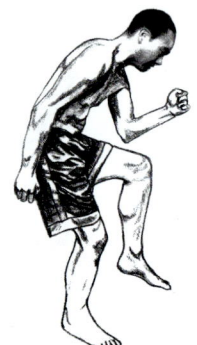
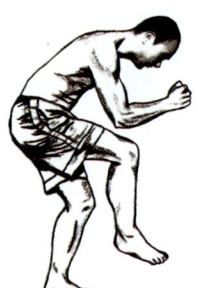
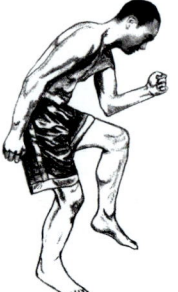

Conclude with Giving Thanks

This is my suggestion for the movements. You may choose to express this emotion in a different way. I find slowing down this eootion to half speed allows the emotion to be felt when you give thanks. It then makes a dramatic conclusion when you return to the normal speed for the Chorus. You may then repeat the Chorus as a final dramatic gesture.

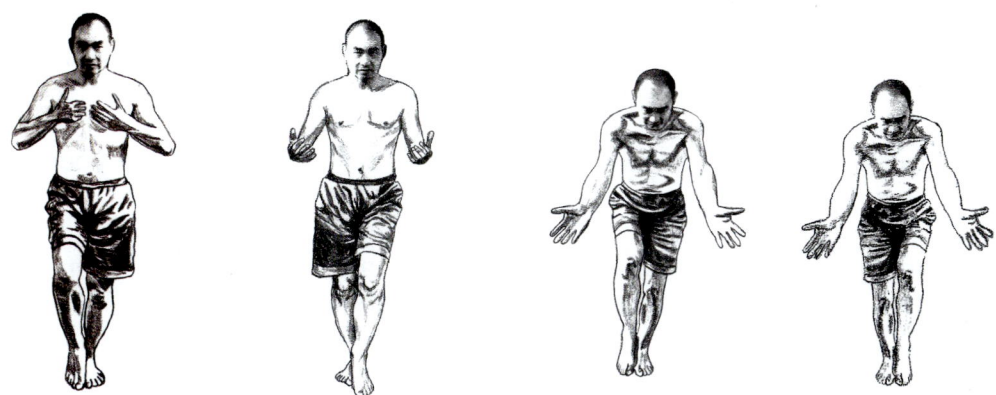

Additional notes

I could not find out if the movements should be right hand and right foot together and left hand and left foot or the opposite sides.

When teaching a seated version to chair-bound pupils, it may be necessary to modify **1. Planting the Seeds** and **6. Picking the Crops** to prevent vulnerable people falling off their chairs.

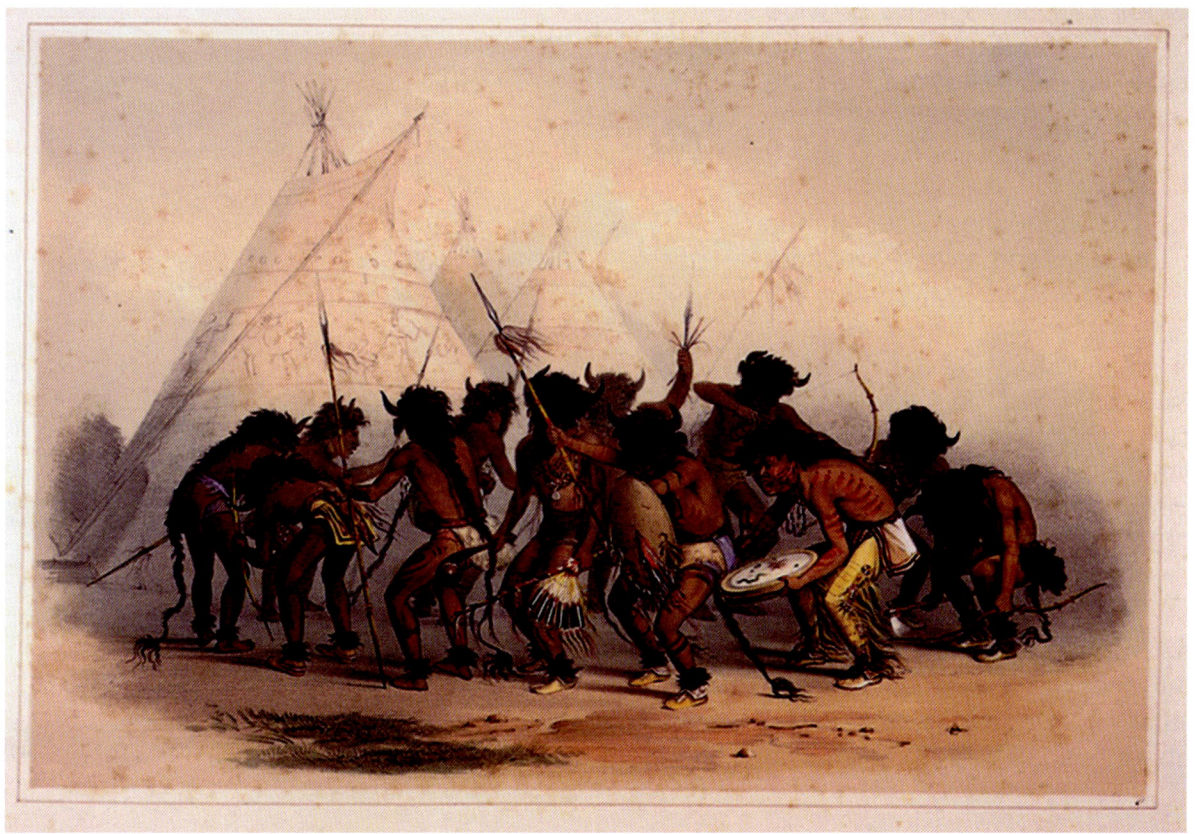

4

1. www.simonheather.co.uk
2. These are likely to have been maize, beans, pepper and squash.
3. Earth, Air, Water and Fire.
4. The Buffalo Dance of the Mandan tribe of North Dakota, painted by George Catlin in about 1860. Permission to include given by Buffalo Bill Center of the West.

Sun Salutations

There are many different versions of Sun Salutations. Swami Saradananda taught this version in one of her monthly workshops in the Booingctoko area. I liked the inclusion of the **Sunburst** and asked her where it came from. She said she had used it in Sun Salutations for a long time and assumed it was standard practice.

You may prefer to work on the three variations for the middle part, between **8** and **13**, before practising the whole of the sequence. There are several variations of these postures and it is necessary to experiment until you find the ones that suit your body type.

When you have decided which variation you prefer, you can incorporate it in your practice or do a few rounds[1] with each variation.

This version is kinder on the shoulders than the traditional Sivananda-style Sun Salutations[1] and is more suitable for those with arthritic and troublesome shoulders.

Preparatory Section

Variation 1

I have used this in the complete sequence on the next page.

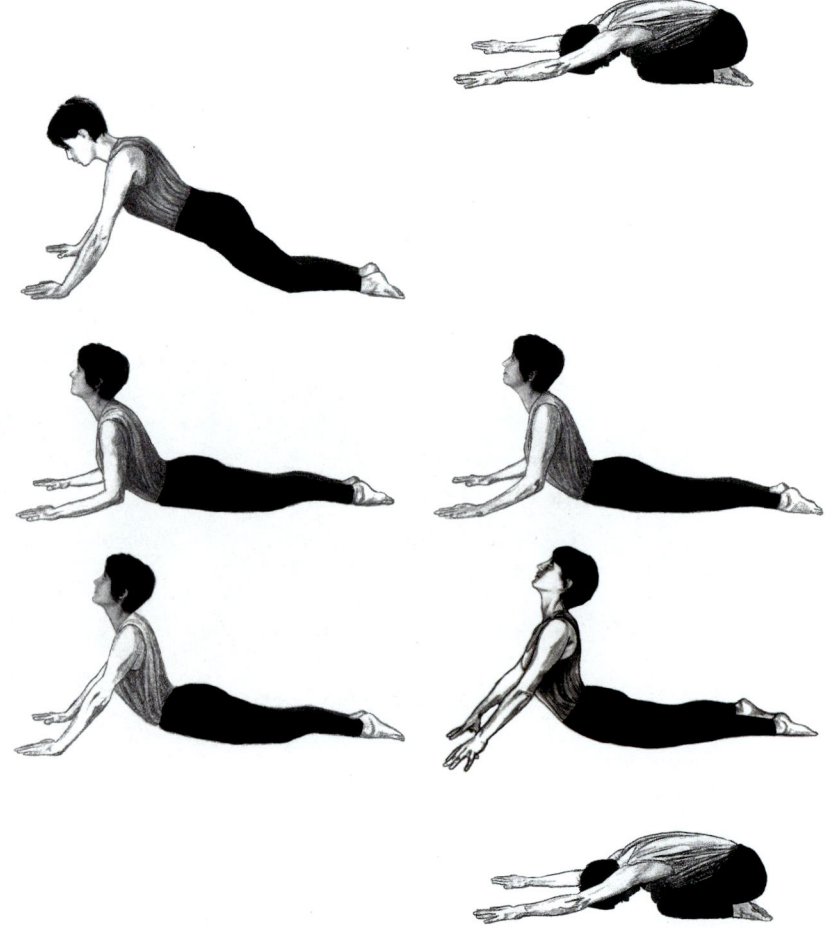

Extended Child's Pose (**10**)
The knees can be together or wide apart. Sit on your feet and push the hips back. Feel the stretch on the lower spine.

INHALE as you slide your hands along the mat and swing forwards (**11**).

EXHALE as you bend the elbows and lower down into **Cobra**. You can experiment to see how much of the abdomen you decide to lower to the floor (**12**).

INHALE up so that your arms are straight and then lean backwards. Alternatively, you can push up on your finger tips (**13**).

EXHALE back into **Extended Child's Pose**.

---

1. A **Round** is the whole sequence twice, once with the right foot backwards in **7** and again with the left foot backwards in **7**.

The hands are further back than in the first variation.

Come into **Extended Child's Pose** with the hands further apart and stretch them as far forwards as you can.

INHALE as you swing your head and shoulders forwards. This time, do not move your hands.

EXHALE as you bend your elbows, keeping them close to your sides. You can experiment with how far you want to lower down.

A. The abdomen can stay fairly high with just the pubic bone touching the floor.
B. You can go half way down.
C. Lower the abdomen to the floor.

INHALE as you push up on the hands and lean backwards.

EXHALE back into **Extended Child's Pose**.

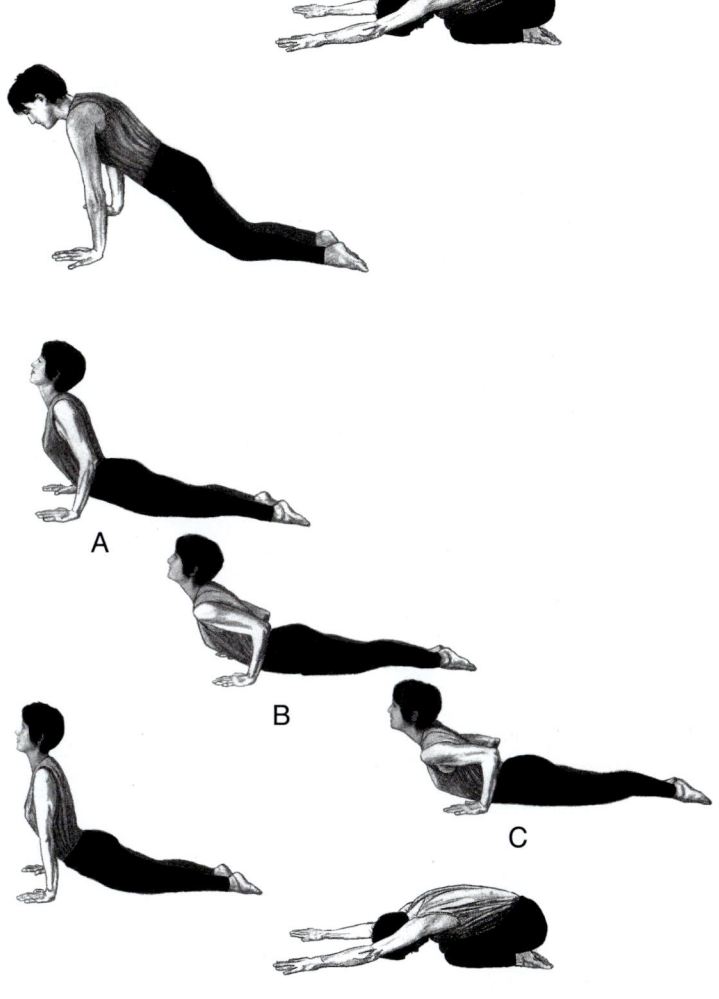

Variation 3

This uses two fewer breaths. From **8,** do not sink back into **9** and **10**. Instead **INHALE** both legs back into **Plank** and **EXHALE** into what I call **Excruciating Posture** (men seem to find it easier than women). It is also called **Four-Limbed Staff Pose**. **INHALE** into **Backward Plank** before **EXHALING** into **Downward Dog**.

INHALE into **Plank**.

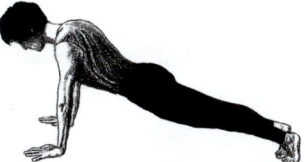

EXHALE into **Excruciating Posture**.
Bend the elbows and lower yourself down as illustrated. The elbows have traditionally been kept close to the sides but I have seen it done recently in videos with the hands turned inwards and the elbows out to the sides.

INHALE as you push up into **Backward Plank**. Lean back as far as you can but only bring the head back if you are sure it is safe to do so.

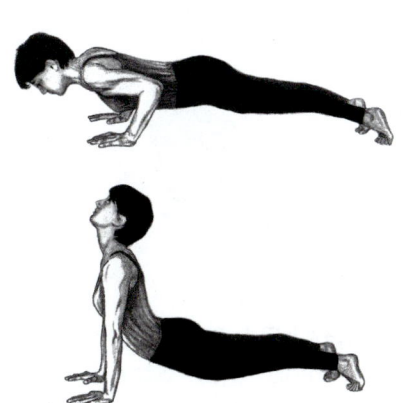

Sun Salutations

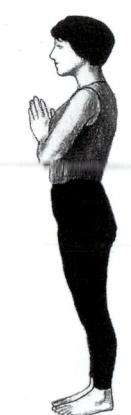

1. Stand with the feet together and the hands in **Prayer**.

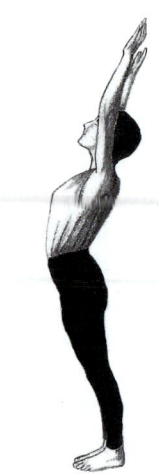

2. INHALE the hands up and back.

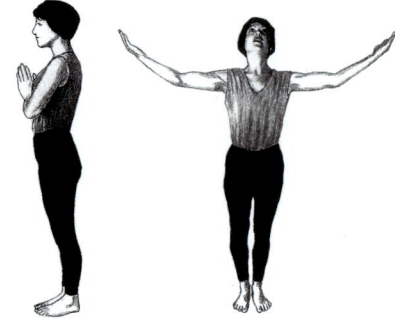

18. Either go straight to **1** or skip to **Sunburst**, **3**, and continue, changing sides at **7**. I prefer to go straight to **3** in the middle of a round and to **1** at the end of each round.

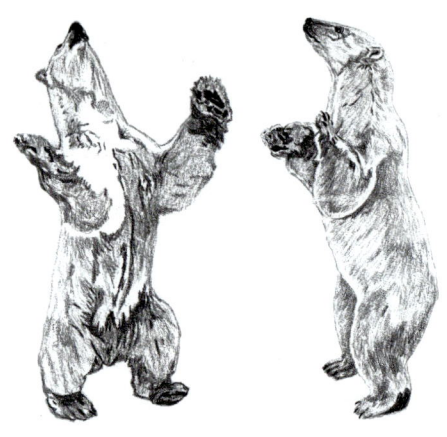

Polar Bear Sun Salutations

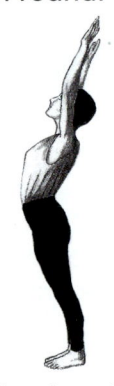

17. INHALE the hands up and back.

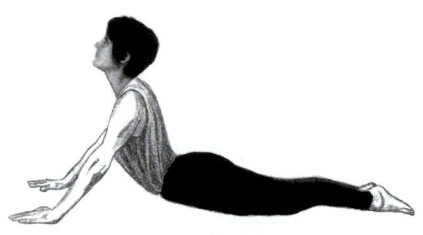

13. INHALE up into **Backward Cobra**.

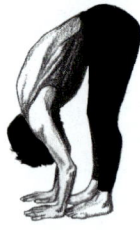

16. EXHALE left foot to right foot coming into **Standing Forward Bend**.

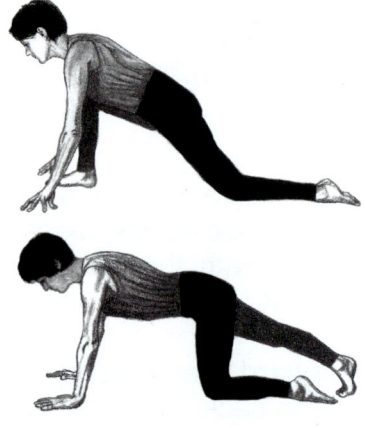

15. INHALE the right foot forward. Some people prefer to put the left knee to the floor first.

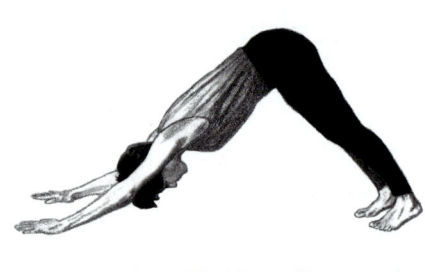

14. EXHALE back into **Downward Dog**.

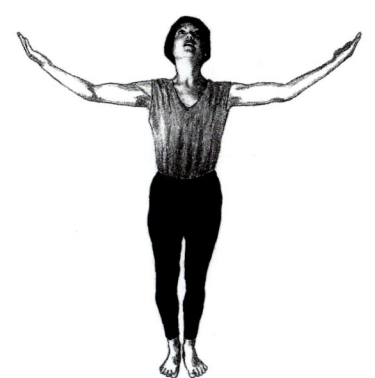 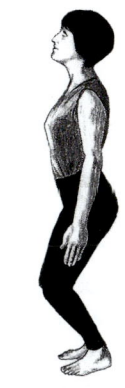 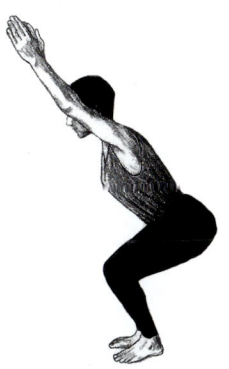

3. **EXHALE** the hands down and out to the sides with a **Sunburst**. Open your mouth and **EXHALE** with a **Ha Breath**. This is like a deep sigh. (see page 11)

4. As you start to **INHALE**, bend your knees and lower your hands to the sides.

5. Continue to **INHALE** into **Upward Armchair**. The tail-bone sinks down low. The palms are facing but not touching. Look up at your hands.

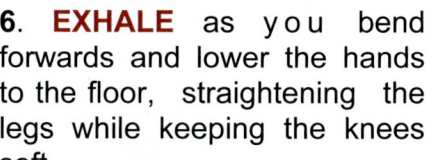

6. **EXHALE** as you bend forwards and lower the hands to the floor, straightening the legs while keeping the knees soft.

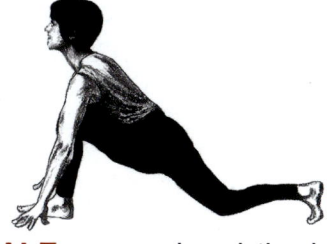

7. **INHALE** as you bend the left knee and step backwards with your right foot, coming onto your toes.

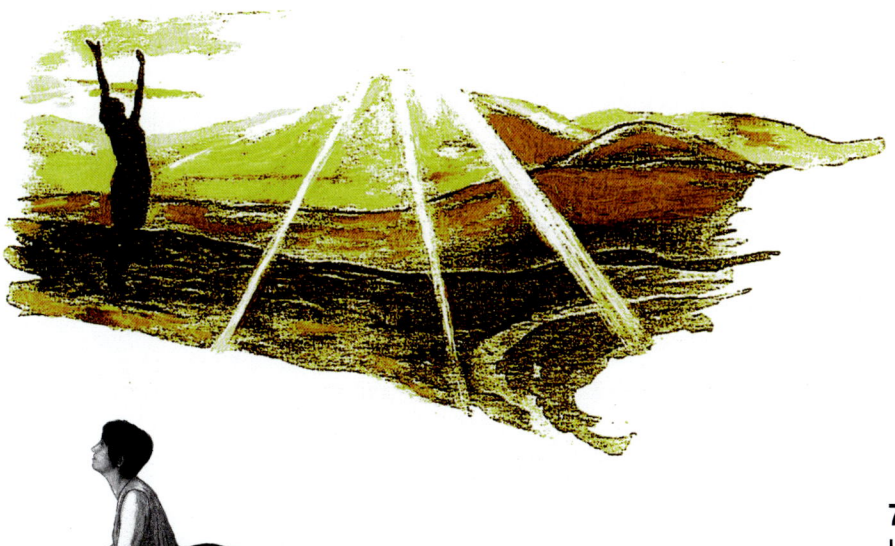

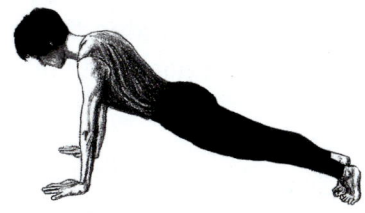

8. **EXHALE** as you step backwards with your left foot, coming into **Plank**.

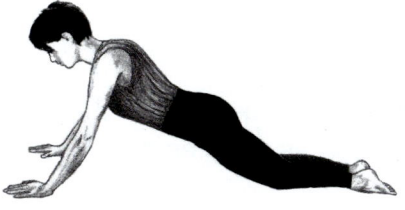

12. **EXHALE** into your chosen version of **Cobra**.

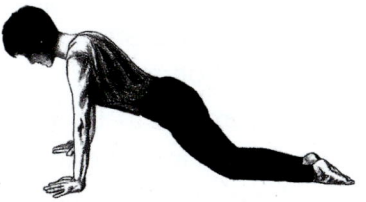

11. **INHALE** as you slide your hands along the mat and swing forwards.

9. **INHALE** as you lower your knees to the floor and flatten your feet.

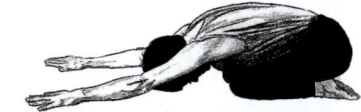

10. **EXHALE** into **Extended Child's Pose**. Stretch the hands forwards and sink the hips back to the heels.

A Final Flourish

This idea comes from a **Liquid Asana** DVD by Micheline Berry. It incorporates well into this version of the **Sun Salutations** as a graceful ending to the practice.

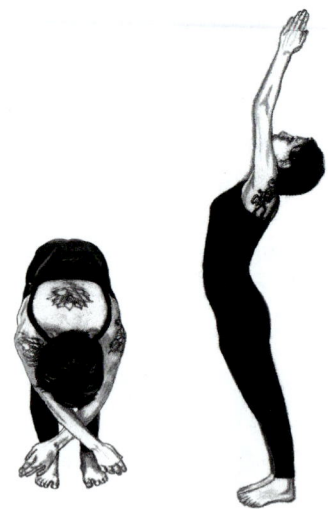

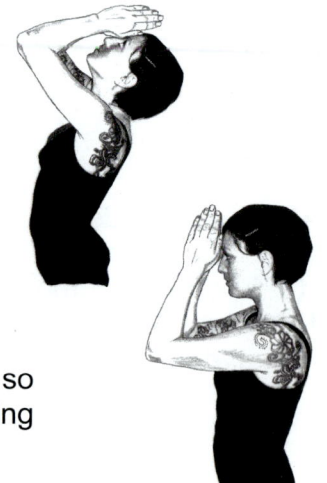

2. Continue to look upwards as you bring your thumbs to the **Third Eye,** the point between the eyebrows.

3. Lower your chin so that you are looking straight ahead.

4. Lower your hands to the **Heart Centre.**

1. From **16,** the **Standing Forward Bend**, swing your hands in front so that the wrists cross over. **INHALE** them out to the sides and up above your head in **Prayer**. Lean backwards and look up at your hands.

Arm Circling Sequence

The breathing instructions are only suggestions. You may prefer to reverse the breathing pattern. For example, in **4,** you may feel like exhaling into **A** and inhaling into **C**. To clear the mind of thoughts and further connect the breath with the movements, you could add counting (as described in **Extending the Breath** on page 10). Alternatively, you can just observe the natural inclinations of your breath.

CAUTION
Those with back problems should be particularly cautious in **2** and **5**. If necessary, consult a medical practitioner before practising them. Stop as soon as there is any discomfort.

SOURCES
1. We did this in a Hot Yoga class at the Wild Lotus Studio in Newbury.
2, 4 and **7A** and **C** are inspired by the DVDs of US-based yoga teacher Micheline Berry.
3. Source forgotten.
5. Tasha from North London-based Tranquility in the City volunteered this idea. My daughter Miriam, who is modelling this sequence, initiated **D**.
6. Reading-based Swami Ambikananda taught this in a workshop.
7B. My daughter, who is a Salsa dancer, said she was taught this in an Indian Dance class during her degree course at Surrey University.
8. Source forgotten.
9. This comes from a video with Eric Schiffman, a US-based yoga teacher.

1. Supine Open Heart Circling

A. Lie on your back with your hands out to the sides and the palms facing upwards. Bend your knees. To make the posture more comfortable, move your hips a little to the right before lowering the knees to the left. Rest your right foot on top of your left foot.
INHALE as you start to circle the right hand above your head.

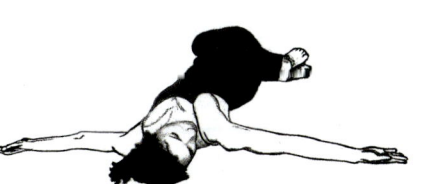

B. **EXHALE** as your hand turns to face downwards as it passes over the left hand. It will rotate upwards as you return to the starting position. Circle the hand slowly at least three times and then change direction.
Change sides and repeat.

Variations

C. You can straighten the right leg.

D. You can place your right knee over the left knee and let the foot rest on the floor.

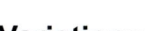

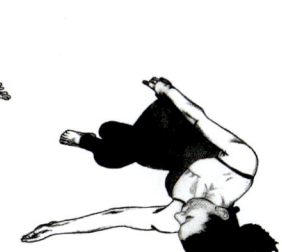

2. Stomach Lock Activation

A. Sit with the knees bent and the feet about 6 inches (15 cm) apart. Lean slightly backwards and bring the hands together with the palms facing upwards.

B. **INHALE** as you stretch the hands forwards. Start to **EXHALE** as you circle them round to the sides and lean backwards. The abdominal muscles will engage to support the spine.

C. Pull your elbows back and into the sides. You may choose to lift the chin, but keep the neck in line with the spine.
Repeat slowly a few times.

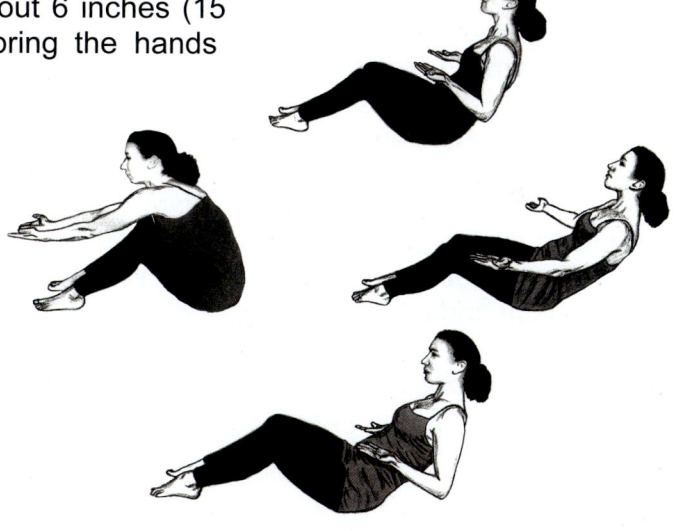

Further Explanation. The drawing in of the abdominal muscles to support the spine is similar to **Uddiyana Bandha**. This is the **Stomach Lock** as described in **The Hatha Yoga Pradipika** (see Glossary). **Ut** and **di** means *to fly up* in Sanskrit. **Bandha** means *lock*. In the ancient text it is practised in a sitting posture. *The lungs are emptied and driven against the upper part of the thorax, carrying the diaphragm along with them*[1]. This was practised with the goal of raising the **Kundalini** (see Glossary). In the above activation, the **Lock** happens naturally, without conscious activation. You may choose to pause briefly in **C** before inhaling forwards.

1. Brahmananda's Commentary from **The Hatha Yoga Pradipika**, Om Lotus Publication. ISBN   0-931546/02/8

3. Ocean Circling

Sit in any comfortable position. Imagine you are swimming in the boundless ocean.

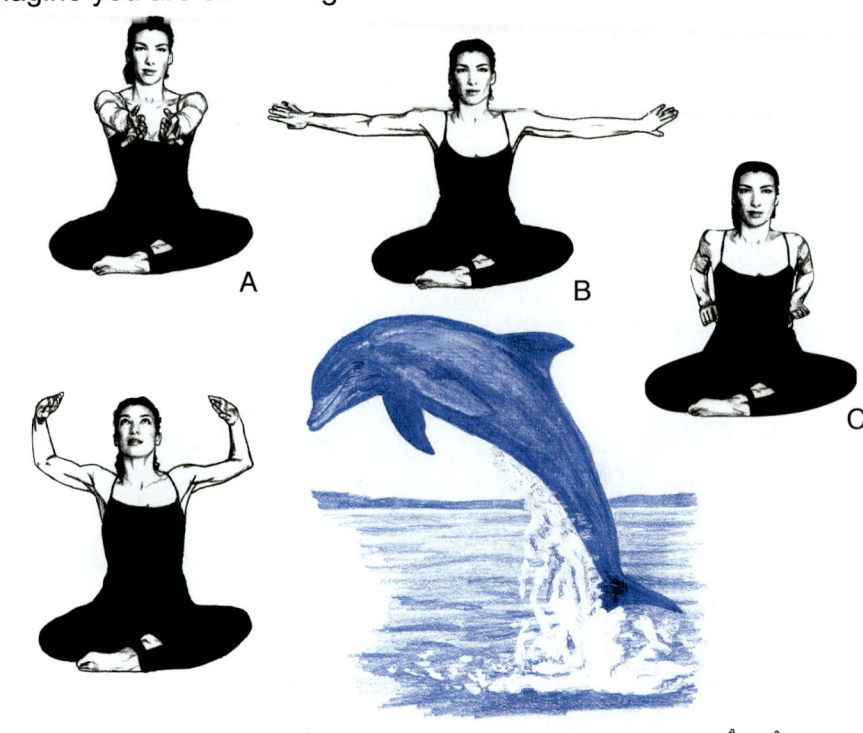

A. Start with the hands close to you at heart level, palms facing downwards. **INHALE** as you stretch the hands forwards with the palms facing outwards.

B. **EXHALE** as you circle the hands wide out to the sides and behind.

C. Return to the starting position but lower the arms to waist level and continue.

D. After repeating at least 3 circles, gradually circle your arms up to heart level and then up to head level.

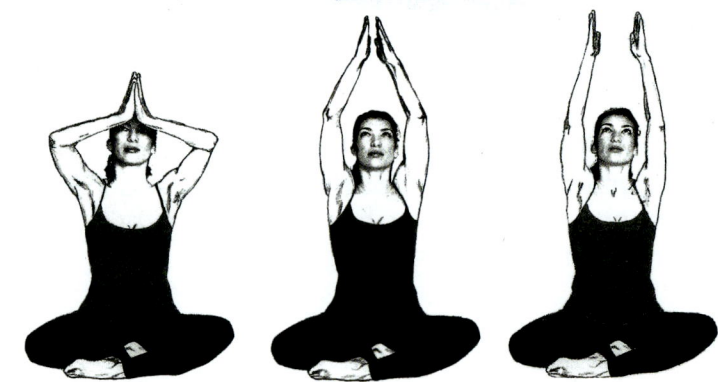

E. Dolphin leaps out of the ocean.
When you feel the time is right, bring your hands into **Prayer**, either in front of your head, as illustrated, or on top of your head. Imagine you are a dolphin leaping out of the ocean. Let your hands leap upwards. Stretch them away and let them separate, as if you were releasing the dolphin to explore freedom.

To conclude, lower your hands to the sides and join them together at waist level and bring them into **Prayer** at the **Heart Centre**. If you are sitting in any cross legged posture, you can reverse the legs and repeat.

4. Heart Opening Standing Rock

Stand with one foot in front of the other, a comfortable distance apart. Bring the hands close to you at heart level with the palms facing downwards.

A. **INHALE** as you bend the front knee, go up on your back toes and stretch the hands forwards. The backs of your hands touch.

B. **EXHALE** as you swing your hands round to the sides and back. Both knees are soft and the heels are down.

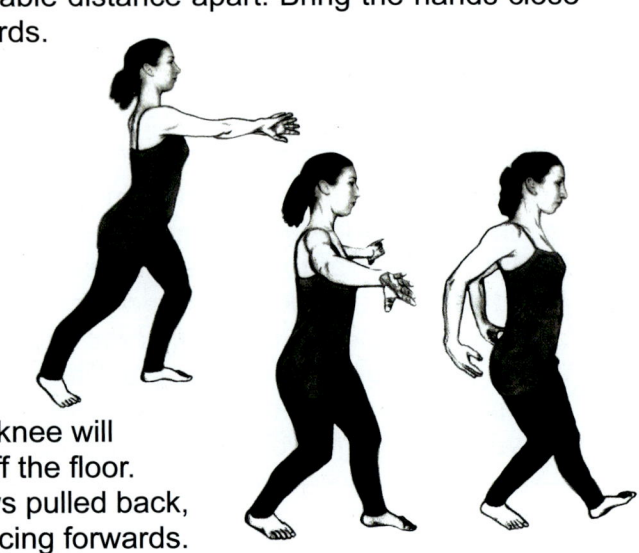

C. As you bring your hands further back, the back knee will bend, the front leg straighten and the toes come off the floor. Pause at the end of your exhalation with the elbows pulled back, the shoulders down and together and the palms facing forwards.
Repeat slowly at least three times and then change legs and repeat.

5. Arm Circling in the Camel Pose

I have illustrated the postures with the tops of the feet on the floor but you may choose to tuck the toes under. Also, you can experiment with the positioning of your knees. You may find some of the variations more comfortable with the knees further apart.

In **B** and **C** you can raise the heel that you are going to rest your hand on and flatten the other foot.

Alternative positions for the feet

A. Kneel with the knees and feet together. Start with the right hand behind your back and the left hand hanging loosely by your side. Begin your circle by moving your left hand across your body to the right. Look at your hand.

Continue to circle round. Follow your hand down and back to the left with your eyes. Make use of your space to make the circle as big as you can.

Allow your hips to circle freely backwards and forwards in reciprocation.

After at least three circles, change direction and repeat.
Change sides and repeat.

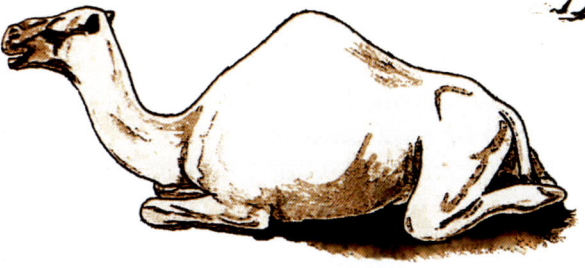

B. Place your left hand on your left heel. Move your hips forward. Circle your right arm as described above. With your hand on your heel, your hips will not be able to move as much as in **A**.
Repeat as above.

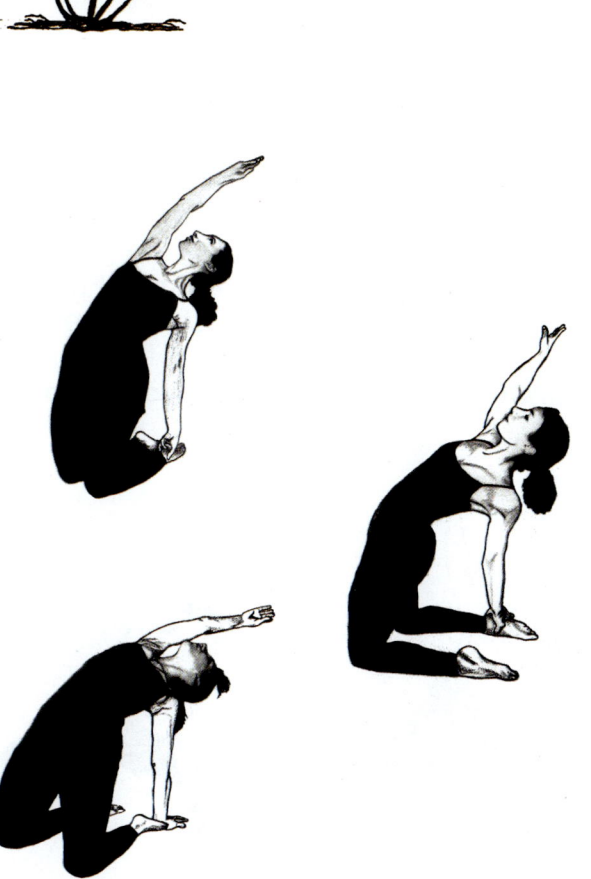

C. Separate the knees and place the left hand on the right heel. Proceed as above.

D. Place your left hand on the floor behind your left foot. The fingers face backwards. Lift your hips and proceed as above.

6. Circle of Light

Start with the feet at least a hip-width apart and the feet turned slightly outwards. Stretch your right hand out to the side with the palm facing upwards. Imagine you are tracing a large **Circle of Light** above you with your hand.

INHALE as you swing it up and over your head. As it swings over to the left, the palm will rotate downwards. **EXHALE** as you stretch it forwards in front.

As you continue to circle the hand round, start to involve the hips. They will naturally move in the opposite direction to your hand. Observe how your weight shifts from one part of your feet to another.

For a variation you can put your passive arm behind your back (as in **7B**).

Change direction and then change hands and repeat.

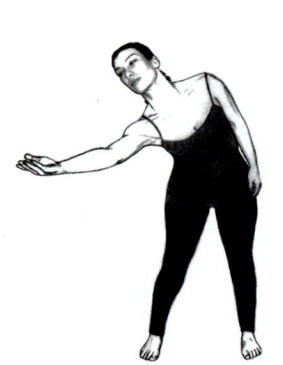 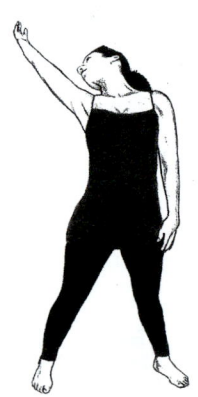 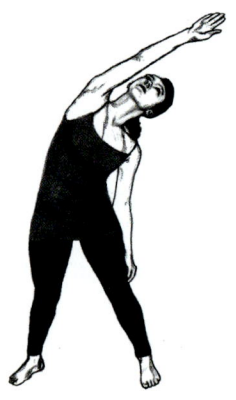

7. Wide Stance Circling

A. Stand with the feet wide apart and turning outwards. Bend your knees, coming into a **Wide Squat**. Place the right elbow on the right knee with the palm facing upwards.
INHALE as you swing the left arm out to the side and up and over your head in a clockwise direction. **EXHALE** as the hand lowers.

After the hand has moved to its lowest point, change the arms over. Place the left elbow on the left knee and circle anti-clockwise with the right arm.

Continue slowly for as long as you choose, gradually deepening the squat.

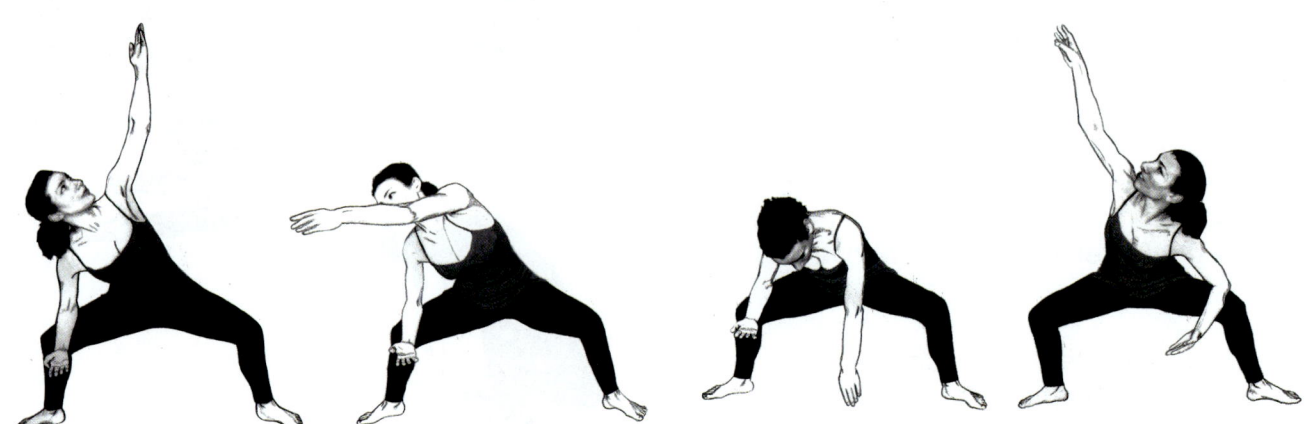

With the feet in the same position, place your left hand behind your back. Start with your right hand fingers touching the floor in front. Circle your hand to the right. Swing it up and over your head and wide to the left.

Try to keep the fingers in touch with the floor for as long as you can. This will alter the shape. Instead of a circle there will be a flat base with a reversed **U shape** on top.

The hips will move forwards and backwards as your hand circles round.

This can also be practised sitting on a chair.
Change direction and then change hands and repeat.

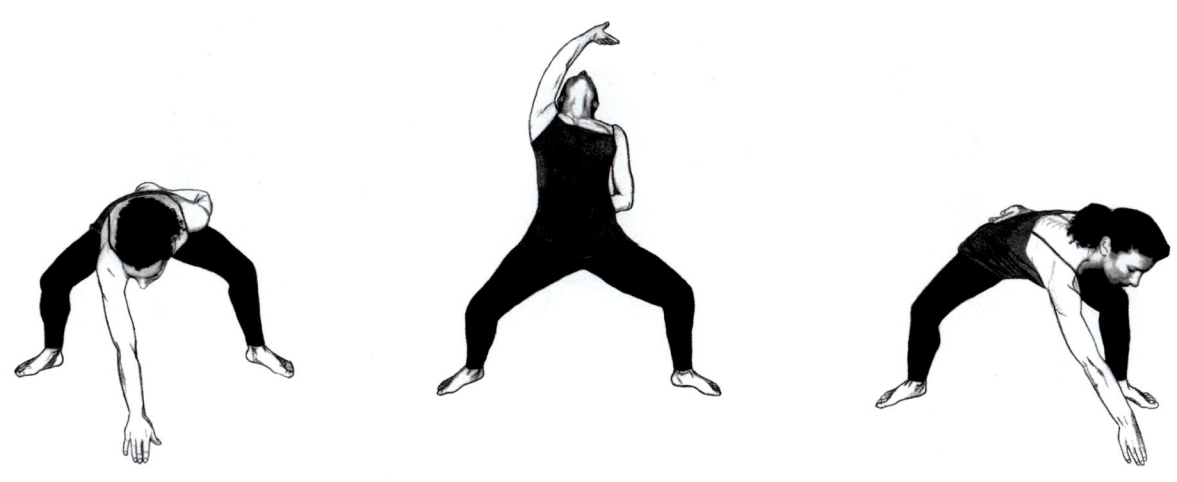

C. Deep Lunge Circling

From the same starting point, turn your right foot to the right and go up on your back toes. Make sure your right knee is above the ankle. Try to make the right thigh parallel to the floor.

Place your right elbow on the right knee with the palm facing upwards. **INHALE** the left hand above your head. **EXHALE** as you swing it in an anti-clockwise direction. Follow the hand round with your eyes.

After at least three rotations, *change direction*. *To change sides*, rotate both feet forward and rest briefly in a **Wide Standing Forward Bend** before turning your left foot to a right angle and going up on your right toes. *Repeat as above.*

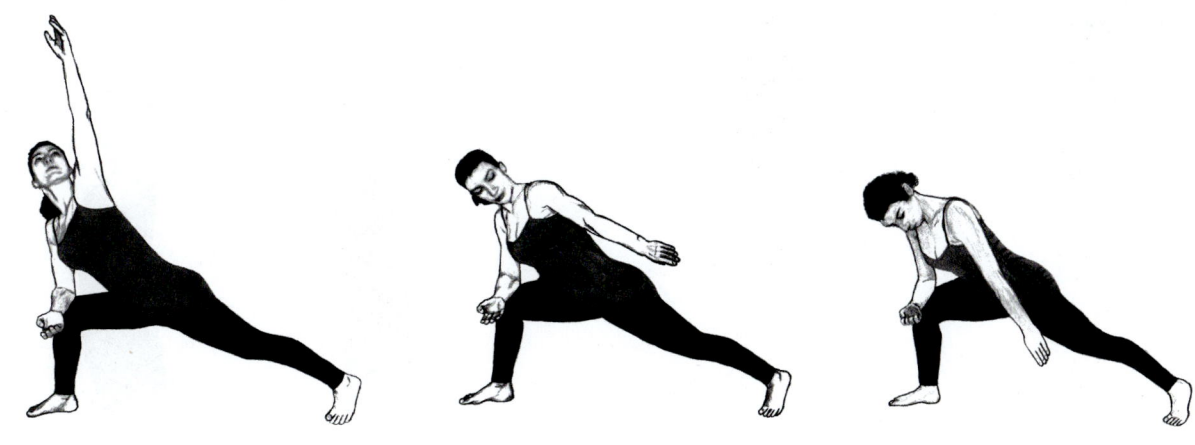

8. Stand with the feet a comfortable distance apart. Catch hold of your elbows with your hands.

EXHALE as you bend forwards. Feel the heaviness of your head. **INHALE** as you circle to the right, bringing the arms above your head.

Continue to circle round to the left, **EXHALING** as you lower the head. Move the hips freely. *Change direction when you are ready*.

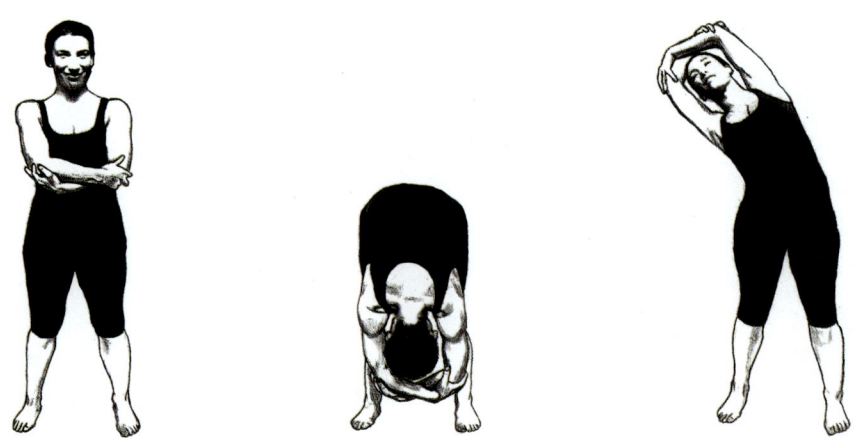

9. Stand with the right foot in front of the left foot. You are going to rock backwards and forwards on your feet and swing the right arm at the same time.

When you swing the arm forwards, lift the back heel. As you swing it back, lower the heel and lift the front toes.

Swing the arm back and forwards a few times to gather momentum. When you feel the time is right, make a full circle with the arm.

Improvise with swinging the arm backwards and forwards and making full circles in either direction.

When you are ready, change sides and repeat.

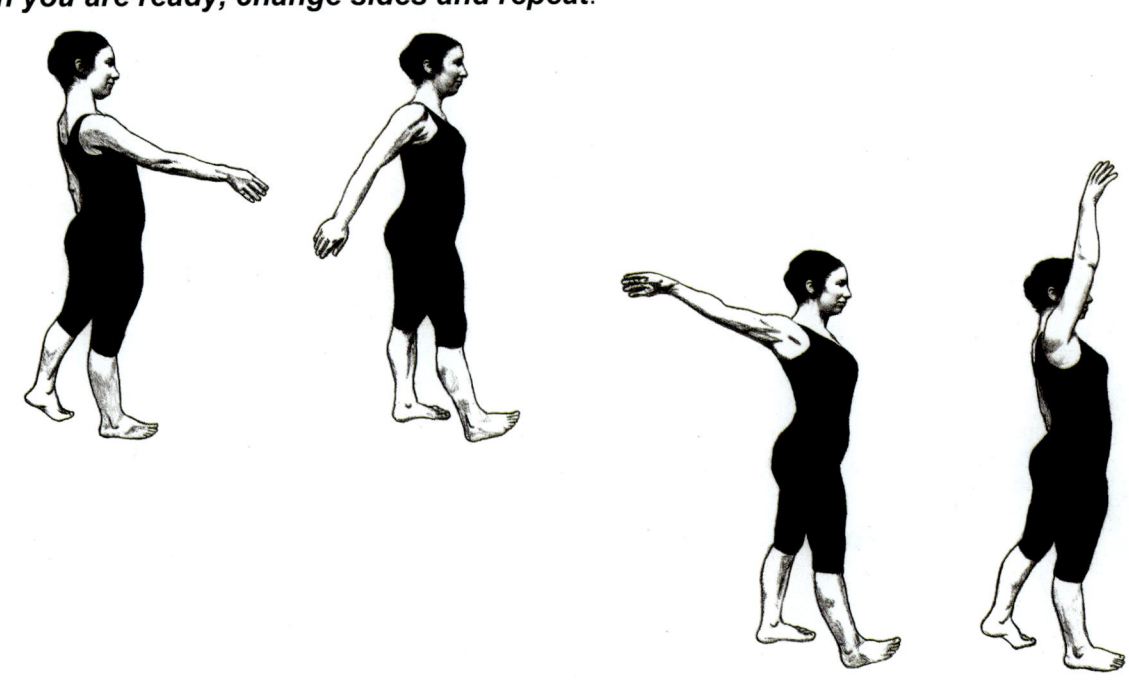

THIS SECTION is inspired by Sophie Gabriel's book *Breathe for Life*[1]. She is not a Yoga teacher but she is familiar with yogic breathing and praises its effectiveness. She teaches correct breathing techniques from the perspective of personal well-being.

She uses the concept of **Nose and Throat Breathing**. This input led me to make the connection between **Nose Breathing** and the **Sympathetic Nervous System**, and **Throat Breathing** and the **Parasympathetic Nervous System**.

In **Nose Breathing** the sensations are felt in the nose. In **Throat Breathing** they are felt in the throat.

Throat Breathing
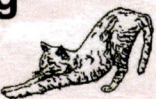
or Ujjayi in Yoga
and Ibuki in Karate

I WILL start with some quotes from Sophie Gabriel's book:

Throat breathing is the kind of breathing that happens naturally when good quality deep breathing occurs ... The sound also gives you the opportunity to monitor and observe the quality and duration of your breathing.

When I am teaching someone how to breathe a good quality breath, the first concept I teach is how to throat breath, and I do not continue with the rest of the training until they have grasped it.

Other names for **Ujjayi** are Victorious Breath[2], Ocean Sounding Breath, Psychic Breath (because of its effect on the mind) and I have even heard it called Darth Vader Breath. I have also added Steam Engine Breath and Dozy Dog Breath (after observing that my brother's dog Rolo, a chocolate Labrador, is an excellent ujjayi breather when he is very relaxed).

Although most people do ujjayi naturally when they are sleeping, or concentrating and relaxing deeply, I find that some of my pupils are timid, awkward ujjayi breathers and don't adjust well to producing the sound in class. In contrast some pupils find it so easy and beneficial that they tend to do it to some degree (loudly or softly) for most of the lesson.

I personally find it so beneficial that I make a point of doing it most of the day (you can do it silently but still put the emphasis on the throat) as a way of inducing the parasympathetic nervous system and saving energy.

You sometimes hear of high achievers who only need a few hours sleep a night. There was an obituary in *The Week* magazine (3 November 07) for the spiritual guru Sri Chinmoy. He claimed only to have needed 90 minutes of sleep a night.

As well as being very strong, Chinmoy was extraordinarily prolific, said The Times. Over the course of his life, he is said to have written 1,500 books, 115,000 poems, and 20,000 songs and to have painted an astonishing 200,000 paintings.

Chinmoy entered very deep states of meditation and taught ujjayi breathing to his pupils. His breathing is most likely to have been of a parasympathetic nature most of the time.

Here are some quotes about ujjayi from the *Hatha Yoga Pradipika*[3].

The practice of ujjayi is so simple that it can be done in any position and anywhere ... It helps relax the physical body and the mind, and develops awareness of the subtle body and psychic sensitivity. Ujjayi promotes internalization of the senses and pratyahara[4].

Ujjayi is especially recommended for people who have insomnia and mental tension. It is a must in the yogic management of heart disease. However, anyone with low blood pressure must first correct their condition before taking up the practice.

Method

The original method was making the noise in the throat while inhaling through both nostrils, retaining the breath and then exhaling quietly and slowly through the left nostril. These are slightly simplified quotes from the same version of the *Hatha Yoga Pradipika*.

Closing the mouth, draw in the breath through both nostrils till the breath fills the space from the throat to the heart with the noise. Perform kumbhaka (pause and hold the breath) *and exhale through the left nostril ...*
This is called ujjayi and it can be done while moving, standing, sitting or walking.

During the last century, some yoga teachers discovered the benefits of using ujjayi during sequential posture work. They omitted the pause and made the noise on inhalation and exhalation. This is now the accepted practice in some yoga classes.

The noise is made by gently constricting the opening of the throat and creating some resistance to the passage of air. It cannot be made without engaging the diaphragm. The diaphragm expands downwards to draw the air in through the slightly closed throat.

Some teachers think it causes tension in the throat and avoid it, but if it is done gently, using our natural technique, it should have the opposite effect.

1. Breathe for Life, *Basic Health Publications, Inc. ISBN 1-59120-002-4*
2. Ujji is the root which means 'to conquer' or 'acquire by contest'.
3. *From the* Hatha Yoga Pradipika. *Commentary by Swami Muktibodhananda Saraswati,
under guidance of Swami Satyananda Saraswati. Bihar School of Yoga. No ISBN.*
4. *The fifth stage in Patanjali's Eight Limbs of Raja Yoga.
It is the process of disconnecting from the outside world and taking the senses inwards before concentration and meditation.*

Tone your Arches

Mara Musso talked about the arches of the feet in an Astanga workshop. She speculated about how our small feet manage to support the much larger body and our wide range of movement. We decided it was the energy created by the three arches in each foot that made them so efficient.

She elaborated that there is a long arch on the inside, a shorter one on the outside and one going across the ball of each foot. We lifted our toes and spread them out a few times to activate them and increase our awareness of them.

This influenced me to develop a short sequence for my pupils. Eventually, you should keep the toes up and wide, without lowering them between **3** and **7**. However, you may need to have a rest between **4** and **5** when you first practise this sequence.

1. Stand with the feet slightly apart and your hands by your sides. Lift your toes as high as you can and spread them out wide. Lower the little toes to the floor and follow with the others, keeping them wide apart. ***Repeat x3.***

2. The **Forward Tilt**. With your toes still wide apart, press them into the floor and tilt forwards. Keep the spine straight. **x2**.
Repeat once more, this time with your heels coming slightly off the floor. Tilt a little further forwards.

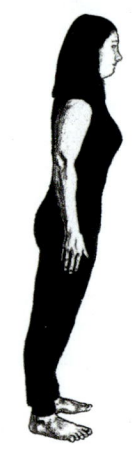

3. Lift your toes high and wide and hold them there. Curve your right arm over your head and stretch the elbow up towards the ceiling, creating a stretch up your right side. Move your hands down to the left. ***Hold for a few breaths and repeat on the other side.***

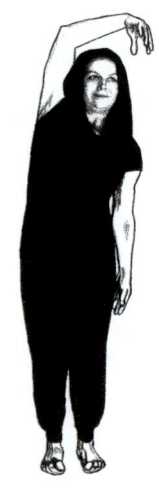

4. Place your fingers on your shoulders. **INHALE** as you move your shoulders and elbows back, expanding the chest. The head can tilt back a little if it is comfortable. **EXHALE** as you round your back and bring your elbows together in front. The chin tucks in. **x3.**
Now lift your left elbow up and back. Look to the left and twist round a little. ***Hold for a few breaths and repeat on the other side.***

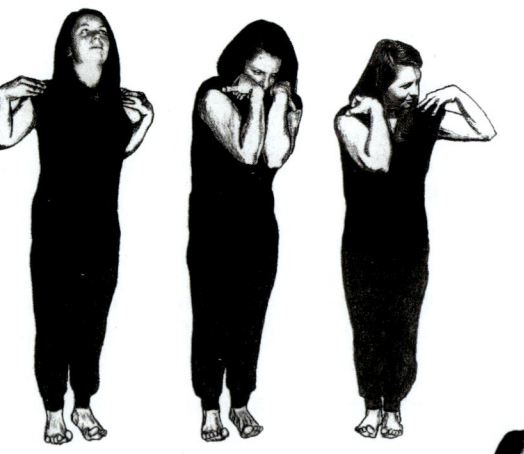

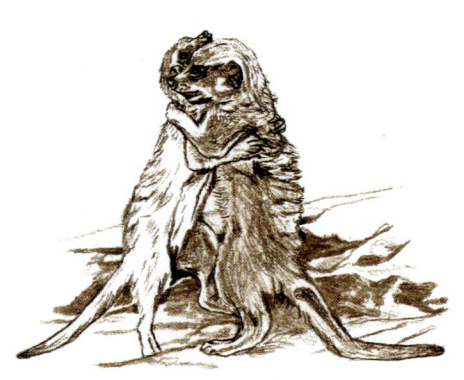

5. Place the heels of your hands in the hollow above your waist. Stretch your head up towards the ceiling and then twist round to the right. ***Hold for a few breaths and repeat on the other side.***

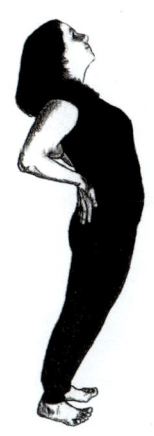

C. Lean backwards slowly and with care. Expand the chest and let the head fall back if it is comfortable. *Hold for a few breaths.*

7. Move into **Fierce Pose**. Bend your knees and stretch your hands above your head in **Venus Lock**. *Hold for as long as you comfortably can. Lower your toes and shake out your legs and feet.*

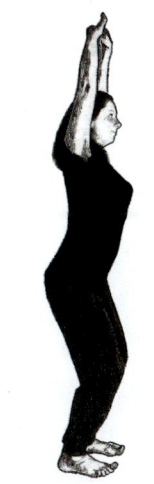

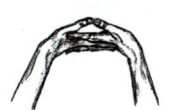

Venus Lock

Relax and shake out your feet.

8. Place a block between your thighs and move your feet closer until you feel the **inner arches** lifting.
Now repeat the whole sequence again keeping the block in place throughout. This will further activate the arches. Pause if you need to and rest the feet before continuing.

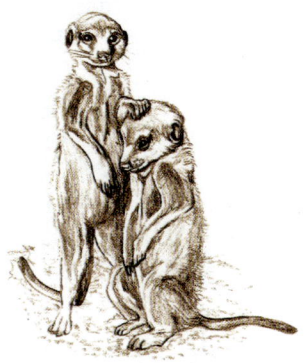

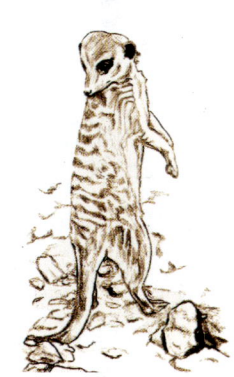

More information about the arches

Feet are important due to their weight-bearing function. Yoga practice places great importance on the role of the feet.

The foot has three arches. These arches are crucial in giving the feet flexibility, absorbing stress, adapting the feet to different surfaces and distributing the weight of the body. These arches play a vital role in yoga practice because they influence the foundations and alignment of the rest of the pose.

1. The medial longitudinal arch runs along the inside of the foot, from the big toe side of the foot to the heel. This arch doesn't touch the ground and is most involved in the weight-bearing function of the foot.
2. The lateral longitudinal arch runs along the outside of the foot. It is mostly involved in propulsion and it does touch the floor.
3. The transverse arch runs across the mid-foot from outside to inside. This arch also provides support and flexibility to the foot.

In standing, a general rule for most yoga poses is that half of the weight should fall on the heel while the other half is divided over the ball of the big and little toe. In standing poses we must try to keep the arches engaged. When you keep the arches engaged correctly, it creates a solid foundation for the rest of the pose.

Journey to the Heart Mudra Sequence

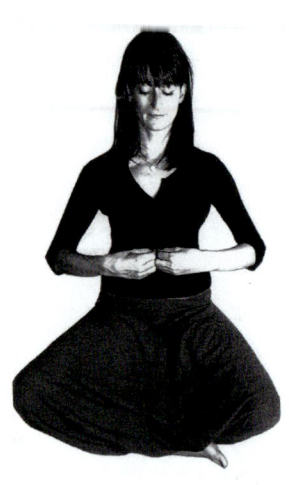

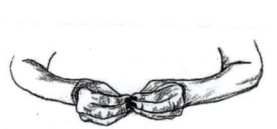

1. Bring the thumbs and fingers of each hand together.

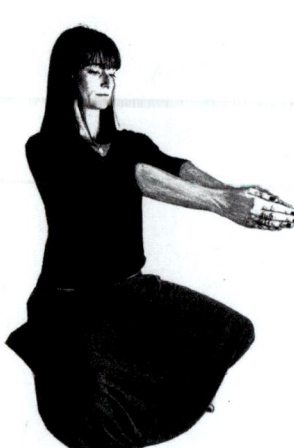

2. Extend the hands forwards with the palms touching.

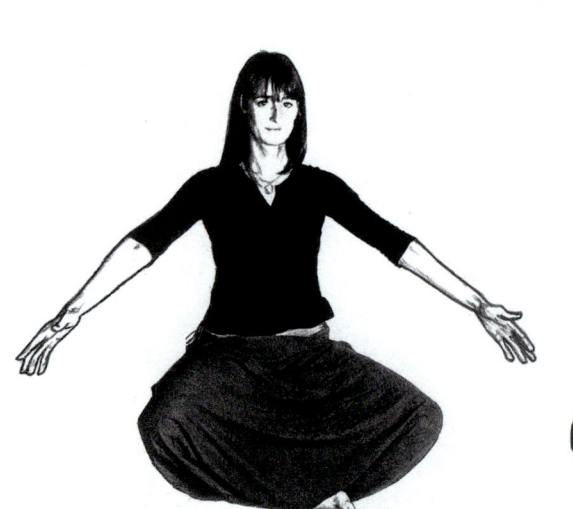

11. Lower the hands.

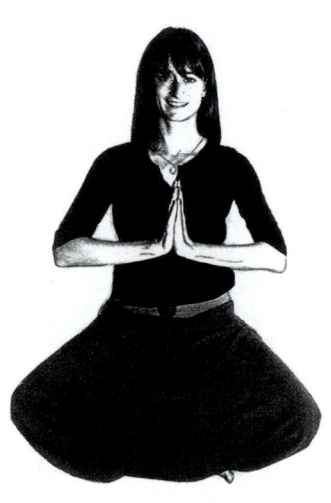

12. Bring the hands into **Prayer** at the **Heart Centre**.

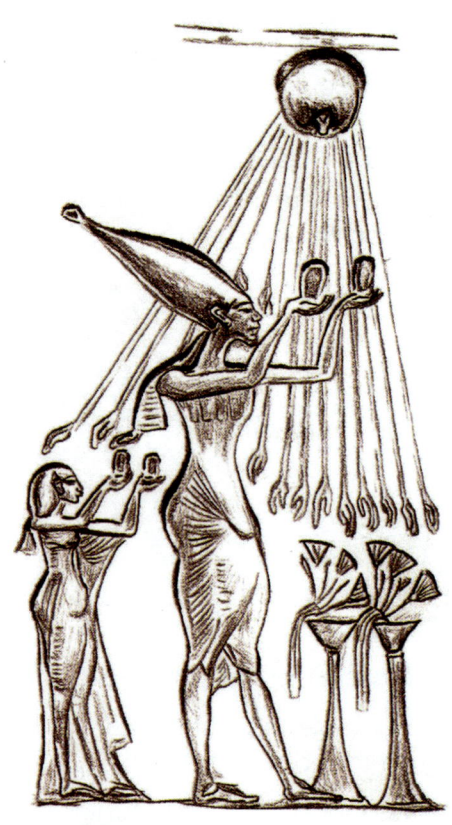

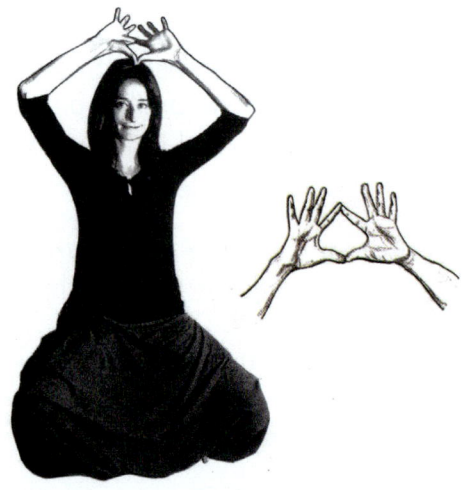

10. With the thumbs touching, bring the index fingers together forming a triangular shape. Lift the mudra above your head with the palms facing upwards.

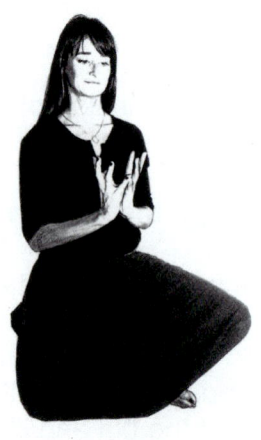

9. Return to **7**.

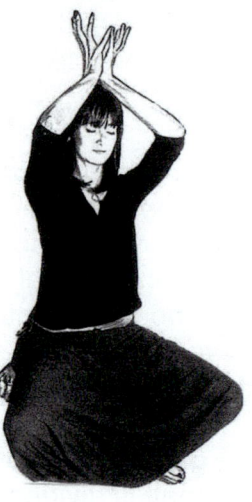

8. Lift the mudra to the top of your head.

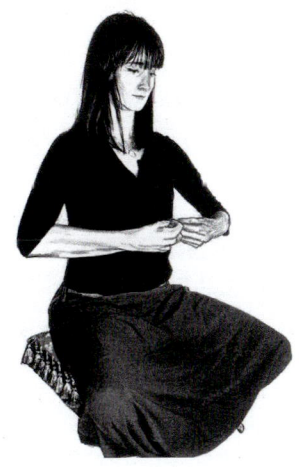

3. Bring the hands back, returning to **1**.

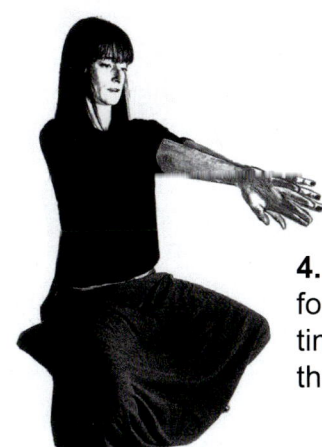

4. Extend the hands forwards again, but, this time, with the backs of the hands touching.

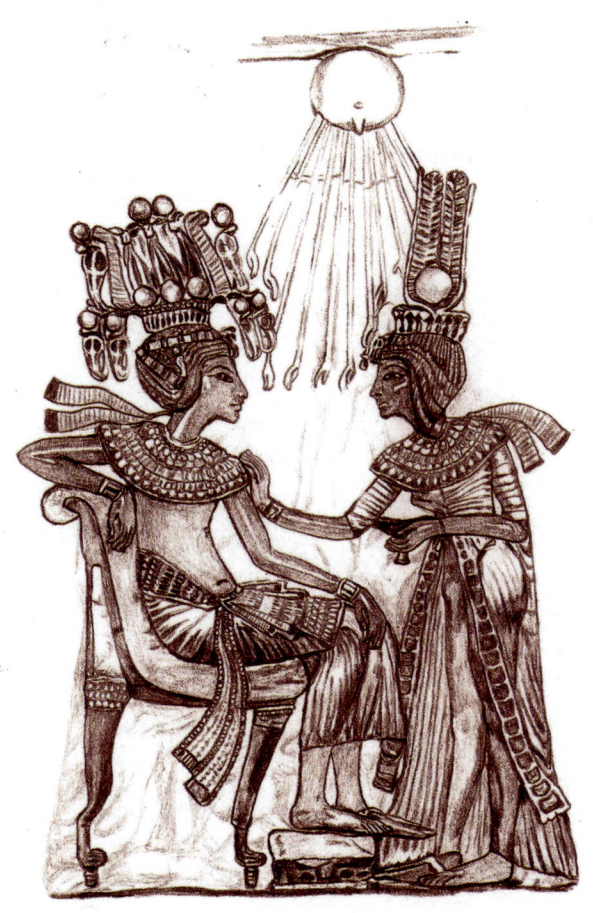

Hands shining from the Sun's Rays
in Egyptian Art
Find more information on page 48

5. Bring the left hand back with the thumb down and the palm facing forwards.
With the fingers together and bent, clasp the right fingers inside the left fingers.
The right palm faces inwards and the thumb is up.

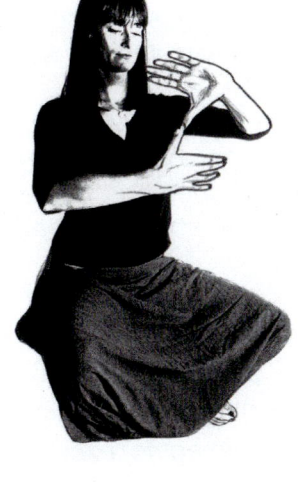

7. With the thumbs still touching, bring the heels of the hands and the little fingers together (as in the top of page 47) Open the fingers out wide.

6. Separate the hands and stretch out the fingers, keeping the palms in the same direction. Let the thumbs touch in the middle.

Journey to the Heart Mudra Sequence

I was introduced to Mudra Sequencing at a workshop with Sue Baynham Evans at the British Wheel of Yoga Congress, 2015. She taught us the sequence she had learnt from Annie Jones on a Dru Yoga weekend in Wales.

By the time I taught it to my pupils it had evolved considerably. My pupils loved it and I had already illustrated my version by the time I finally managed to contact Sue and find out more about it. She told me it was the **Heaven and Earth Mudra Sequence**, so I joined the Dru Yoga Video library and watched it.

My third-hand version is so different from the original that I have renamed it, but I remain grateful to Dru Yoga for the subtle and profound inspiration.

You can practise your Mudra sequences standing, sitting, or moving. However, as your concentration will be directed to your hands, you may prefer to be less aware of the rest of your body. You are likely to find this easier if you are sitting. Please follow the advice about **Sitting for Meditation** on page 102.

Mudra Sequencing and the Breath
When I first learnt and taught this sequence, I let my breath naturally follow and flow with the hand movements. I observed it but didn't try to control it. It is indeed a pleasure to feel your full awareness lightly and subtly concentrated in your hands.

Later I taught this sequence a few times at the beginning of a class to connect to the breath. We **inhaled** the hands into **Prayer, 2**, and **exhaled** them back into **3**, and continued like that for the rest of the sequence. You finish up **inhaling** into **10**, **exhaling** the hands down to the sides, **11**, and **inhaling** them up to the **Heart Centre**. It worked out well but it forms an impression that is difficult to forget. It may be difficult to return to your original sublime feeling as you will want to repeat the breathing pattern. You can experiment and discover which method you prefer.

You may prefer to find out the names of the mudras and their interpretations after you have fully experienced the practice. Words and names can sometimes get in the way and distract you.

A Brief Introduction to Mudras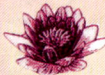

Sources of Information
Presenting Mudra sequences for this book introduced me to a whole new magical world. Some of the information in this section comes from books, mainly **The Healing Power of Mudra** by Rajendar Menen, **Mudras; Yoga in your Hands** by Gertrud Hirschi and **Mudras for Modern Life** by Swami Saradananda. The rest comes from the boundless ocean of information on the Internet about Mudras. I could have written much more but have decided to give you a brief introduction and references to the websites and videos I found most inspiring.

Danielle Prohom Olson writes in **Coming to Grips with the Divine: The Sacred Language of the Hand:**

> In the past few years my hands have taken on a life of their own. During yogic and meditative states, an external/internal energy begins to pour into my palms, compelling my hands to form basic shapes and gestures. Sometimes it feels like my hands and fingers are being pulled by a force, other times it feels as if they are seeking to express something, embody something – but what?
> So in the quest to better understand what was happening, I began to research everything I could find out about the hand. And what I discovered was revelatory.

Her web page (www.bodydivineyoga.wordpress.com/tag/mudras/) contains information about recent scientific research studies on hands. Here are a few gems from it:

> Neural imaging experiments on mudras have demonstrated not only their ability to activate specific parts of the brain, but to alter brain waves and create specific physiological states…

> Denis and Walter found the natural energy in the palms was similar to the two different energies that exist in all magnets. By clasping the hands together in prayer, or Anjali Mudra as it is called in yoga, a 'closed loop' or a 'closed circuit' is formed. Energy flows through this circuit from right hand palm (positive) to left hand palm (negative) enhancing the flow of electrical energy within the body. Interestingly, this is similar to the Taoist view of the left hand as conducting yin energy and the right hand, yang energy…

Research conducted in Japan demonstrated that practitioners of healing and martial arts techniques… were capable of emanating extraordinary large strong pulsating magnetic fields from the palms of their hands, about 1,000 times stronger than normal human bio-magnetic fields

Experiments by John Zimmermann with a highly sensitive Superconducting Quantum Interference Device measured increased magnetic field emission from the hands of psychic healers hundreds of times stronger than normal body activity.

… most amazing are the countless experiments demonstrate that this 'field emission' is capable of altering enzyme activity in cells, changing the Ph level in water, and increasing the growth rate of plants.

Here are other relevant sources: The YouTube video, **Sacred Hand Mudras** by **David Fuess**, gives inspiring instructions about Mudras and includes **Baba Hari Dass** (born in 1923) moving from one mudra to another while the Gayatri Mantra plays in the background. Other Teachers to whet your appetite further are **Vijay K Bansal**, www.mudravigyan.com and **Mr. Parvez Daruwala**.

If you would like somebody singing in the background while you practise the **Gayatri Mudra Sequence**, the obvious choice is the YouTube video by **Deva Premal**. It lasts for two hours.

General Information

   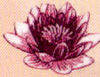

As you position your fingers in different ways, you can influence the flow of energy around your body. When you press the fingertips, or join them together, pressure points and Meridians[1] are activated. The ancient yogis explored the science of hand mudras and mapped out their conclusions. Detailed descriptions can be found in the ancient texts[2]. They considered mudras to be powerful tools for healing.

In his book, **The Healing Power of Mudras**[3], Rajendar Menen offers 20 mudras that have been shown conclusively to heal. He suggests holding some of them for 45 minutes or three times a day for 15 minutes. Other sources suggest 25 minutes or different durations for their suggested mudras.

Many people develop a great love for the Gayatri mantra. It becomes an essential part of their lives. Here are some examples of this.

At the 30-year celebration of the beautiful Mandala Yoga Ashram in South Wales in 2016, we sang it continuously around a fire for four days. We took it in turns to keep it going through the night.

My pupil Josie, who is modelling the **Floor and Wall Sequence**, has a great resonance with the Gayatri mantra. She painted the picture on page 48 for me as a Christmas present. It is 30 inches square. It hangs proudly on the wall in my yoga room.

A friend I met on a Sivananda Sadana Intensive course in France in 2007 has studied in India with a disciple of Swami Rama, intermittently, for the past few years. Under his tutelage, he uses a mala (a string of 108 beads to help him count) and makes many daily repetitions of the mantra. In the first month of practise he made 125,000 repetitions and he was instructed to work towards 300,000. Now he is working towards 1,000,000 repetitions. When I heard from him at Christmas 2016, he had made 500,000 repetitions and so he was half way there.

He says, *'The purpose of the gayatri is deep purification. The practice is daily and the goal to reach 1,000,000 repetitions. The amount of time that will take will depend on your capacity and amount of time available'.*

He was told by his teacher to keep the practice secret and this is the briefest of outlines. Do not attempt this at home. Some of the advanced yoga practices should only be done with the guidance of an experienced teacher and in a peaceful, natural environment. The modern life-style and environment are not conducive to the intense transformational states that are the result of these practices.

1. Meridians are the same as Nadis in Yoga. They are energy channels. They have no membranes and cannot be seen but can be traced in little spiral granules of Hyaluronic Acid (HA).
2. They are found in **Tantra Shastra, Upasana Shastra, Nritya Shastr**a and several other ancient texts.
3. First published by Singing Dragon in 2010. Other publications have followed.

The Gayatri Mudra Sequence

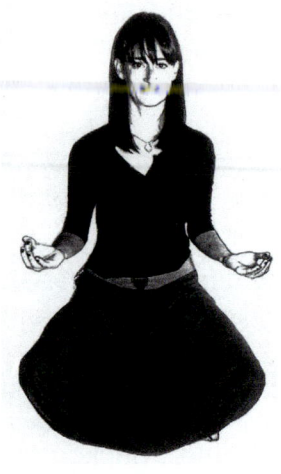

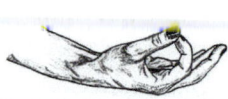

Om

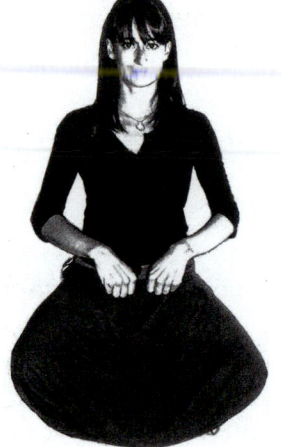

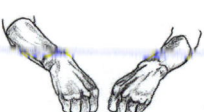

bhur
body
earth

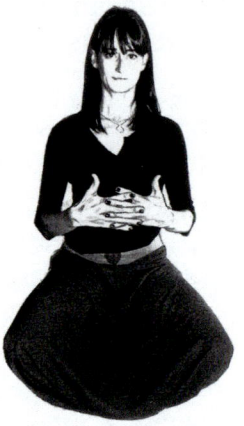

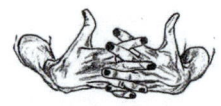

bhuvah
mind
sky

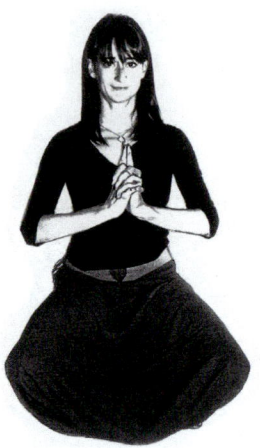

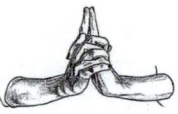

swaha
spirit
heaven

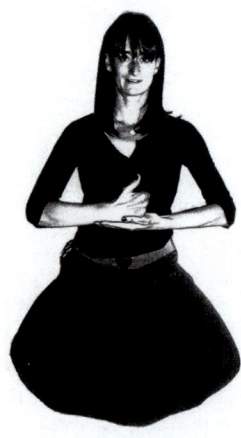

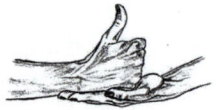

tat
that

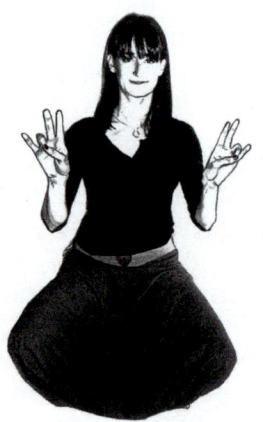

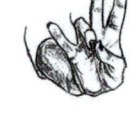

savitur
God of the sun

The Gayatri Mantra
Please note, variations are found in the spelling of this mantra.

Om bhur bhuvah swaha

Tat savitur varen(i)yam

Bhargo devasya dimahi

Dhiyo yo nah prachodayat

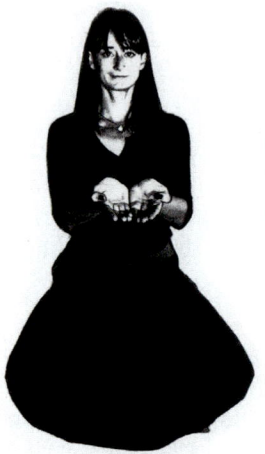

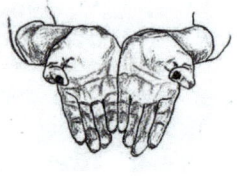

varenyam
we venerate

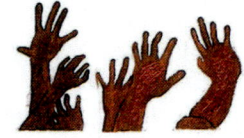

There are many different melodies for the Gayatri Mantra and there is an improvisatory quality to most. If you are not familiar with one of these melodies, there are lots of different versions on the Internet to choose from. Alternatively, you can say the mantra out loud or internalise it while working through the mudra sequence.

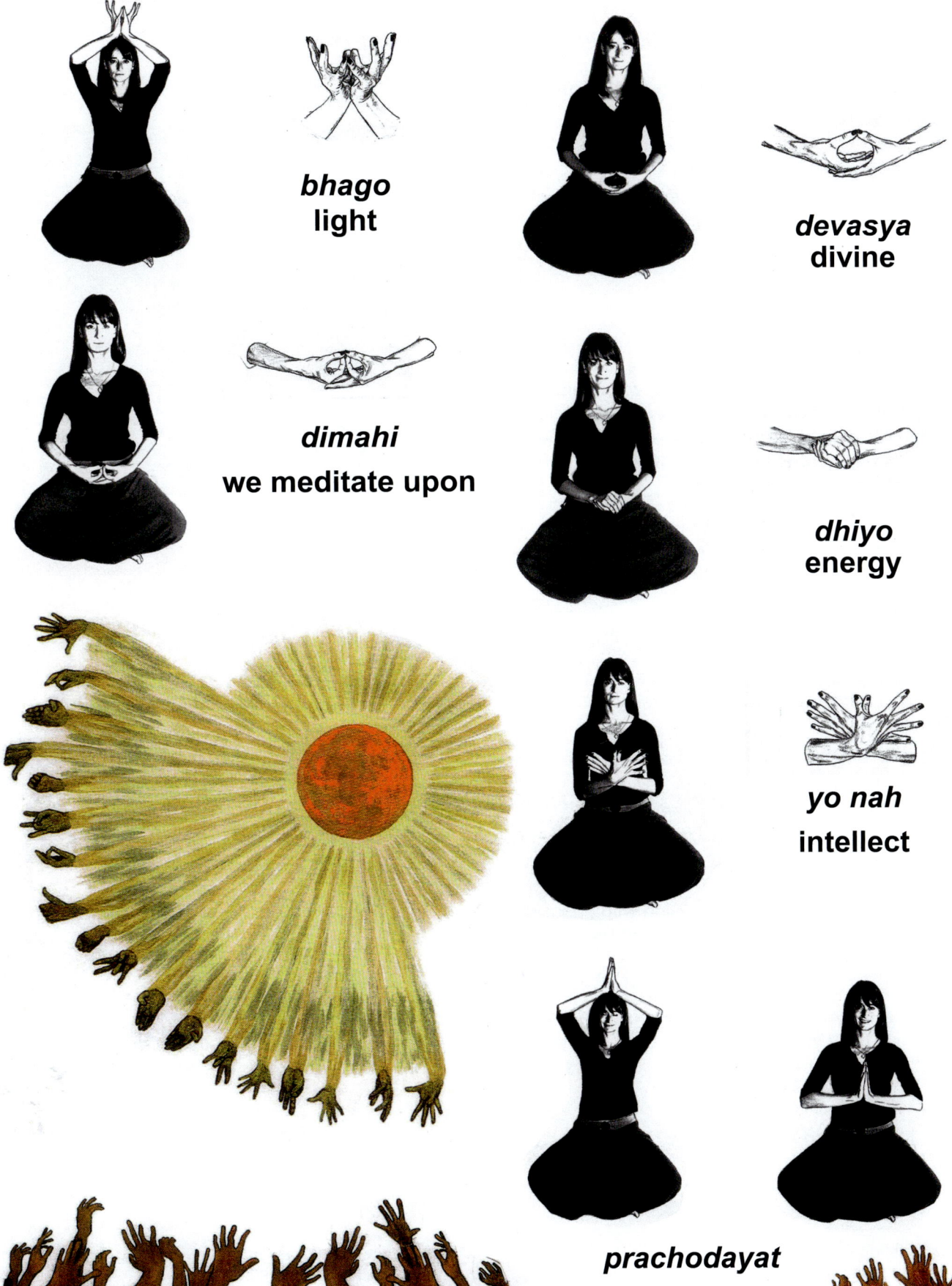

bhago
light

devasya
divine

dimahi
we meditate upon

dhiyo
energy

yo nah
intellect

prachodayat
to inspire us

The Gayatri Mudra Sequence

After my introduction to Mudra Sequencing, I searched the Internet to learn more. I came across a YouTube video of a mudra sequence for the **Gayatri** mantra. It is one of my favourite mantras and the attraction was instant. The lady demonstrating it said she had learnt it from Joseph and Lilian Le Page of Integrative Yoga Therapy at their Enchanted Mountain Centre in Brazil. They kindly gave me permission to include it in this book.

The Gayatri Mantra comes from the ancient Indian text, the **Rigveda**. This is a large collection of devotional hymns and verses written between about 1700 and 1100 BC.

Here are some of the many translations of the Gayatri Mantra

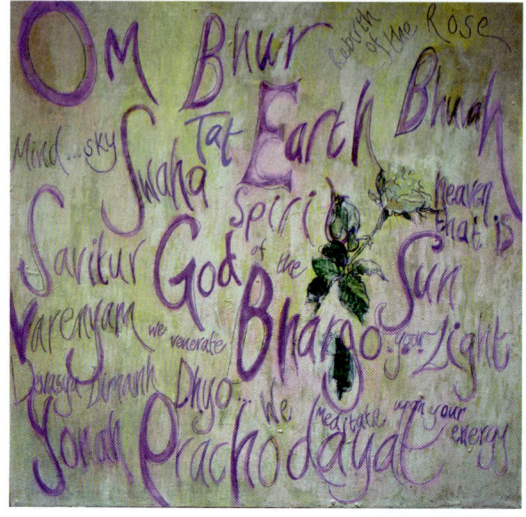

7

1

Om, body mind and spirit (that are expressions of)
That Sun God (consciousness)
That we venerate
May that divine Light which we meditate upon
Inspire our vision and energy.

2

Unveil, O Thou who givest sustenance to the Universe, from whom all proceed, to whom all must return, that face of the True Sun now hidden by a vase of golden light, that we may see the truth and do our duty on our journey to the sacred state.

3

We meditate upon the radiant, divine light of the adorable sun of spiritual consciousness. May it awaken our intuitional consciousness.

4

I meditate on the divine light, the ultimate source of energy that illuminates all life.
May it remove my ignorance, enlighten my mind and impart a perfect understanding of reality.

5

Everything on the earth, in between and above is arising from one effulgent source.
If my thoughts, words and deeds reflected this complete understanding of unity,
I would **be** the peace I am seeking in this moment.

6

O Divine mother, our hearts are filled with darkness. Please make this darkness distant from us and promote illumination within us.

Egyptian Art Work

Page 42, Akhenaten, father of Tutankhamun and Kiya, one of his wives.

Page 43, Tutankhamun sitting on his throne with the hand of his consort/wife on his shoulder.

Aten was the Egyptian Solar God. He was depicted as a sun disc from which the rays ended in extended hands. The sun disc was also encircled by an arc with a rearing cobra symbol.

*The Gayatri has 3 parts: **Praise, Meditation, and Prayer.***
First the Divine is praised, then it is meditated upon in reverence and lastly an appeal is made to the Divine to dispel the darkness of ignorance to awaken and strengthen the intellect. **Sathya Sai Baba**.

The Gayatri mantra helps us wash away karmic impurities and is one of the most powerful mantras for purifying the mind and heart.
Pandit Rajmani Tigunait. PH.D.

1. Translation by Joseph Le Page.
2. William Quan Judge 1893.
3. J. Krishnamurti.
4. From the Dru Yoga book, **Dance between Joy and Pain**.
5. Translation by Donna Farhi from **Bringing Yoga to Life**.
6. From an article by Gyan Rajhans.
7. The painting above is by Josie Simister, 2016.

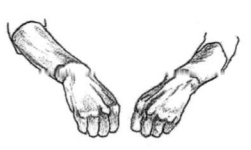 **Adhi Mudra.** The thumb is under the fingers. It opens the upper regions of the lungs, increases oxygen flow to the heart and head areas. It is recommended to reduce snoring.

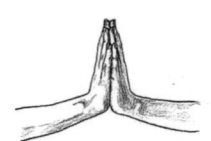 **Atmanjali**, **Anjali**, **Namaska** or **Prayer Mudra**. **Atmanjali** means *Reverence to the Self*. It harmonises the left and right hemispheres of the brain, calms our thoughts and creates clarity.

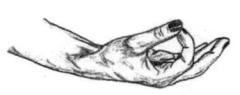 **Chin**, **Jnana** or **Gyan Mudra**. Some sources say it is **Jnana** when the fingers are facing upwards and **Chin** when the fingers are facing downwards. It is recommended for mental and emotional issues[1], and also high blood pressure.

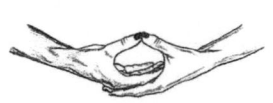 **Dhyana Mudra**. It is the gesture of concentration and meditation. The hands form a bowl or empty space which your mind is mirroring during meditation. It is an invitation to receive wisdom and positive energy.

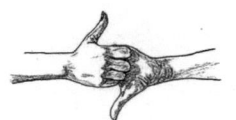 **Ganesh Mudra**. It stimulates heart activity, strengthens heart muscle and opens the bronchial tubes.

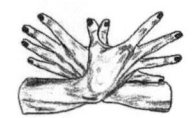 **Garuda Mudra**. It activates blood flow and circulation, invigorates the organs and balances energy on both sides of the body.

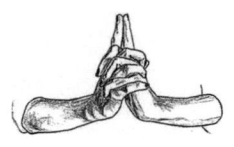 **Ksepana Mudra**[2]. The thumbs are crossed over. It stimulates elimination via the large intestine, skin and lungs and gets rid of negative energy.

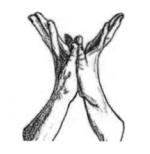 **Lotus Mudra**. It is the symbol of purity. It is associated with the Heart Chakra and receiving and allowing.

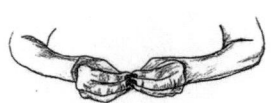 **Mukula Mudra** or **Bird Beak Mudra**. It can be used as a healing mudra if the fingertips are placed on or near the part of the body that needs healing energy.

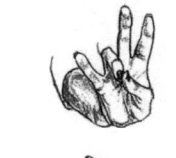 **Prithi Mudra**. It sends energy to the pelvic floor (Root Chakra), intensifies the sense of smell and is good for the nails, skin, hair, joints, and bones.

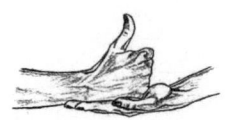 **Shivalinga Mudra**. This is energy charging. It is good for tiredness and depression.

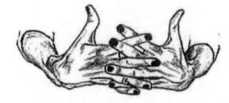 **Vajrapradama Mudra**. It is the gesture of unshakable trust. It is good to do when you lack confidence and feel insecure.

1. Mr. Parnez Darival talks about it in his **Health in your Hands** YouTube video.
2. This is affectionately known as **James Bond** mudra in the Newbury area where I live, after a local yoga teacher started to call it this in her classes.

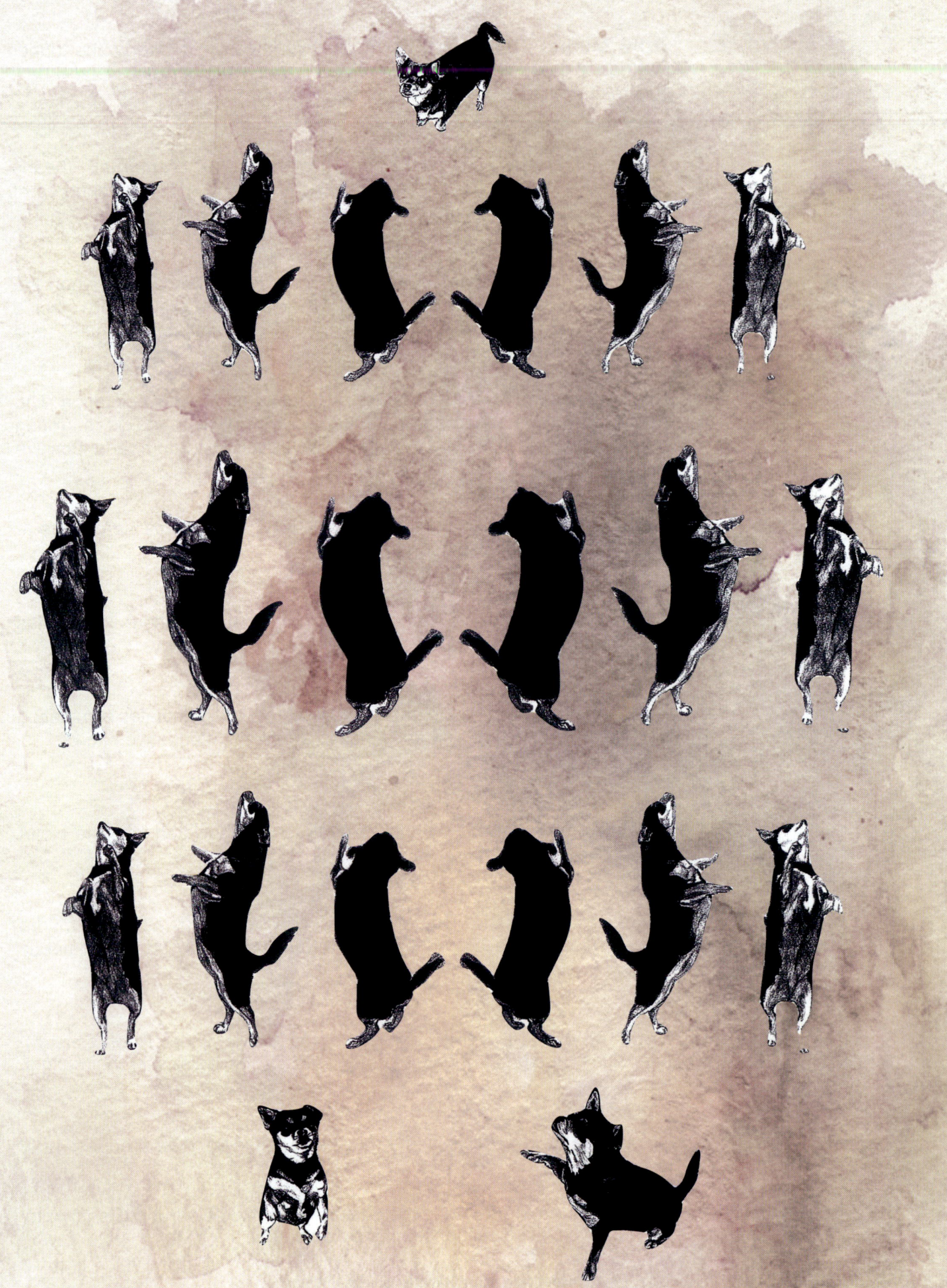

Hanuman's Leap
A sequence with a story

Bob Camp gave me ideas for many sequences in my earlier books. He is still teaching in his eighties in Norfolk.

He sent me his version of **Hanuman's Leap**. I have added detail and more postures, and presented it so that a story can be narrated at the same time as it is practised, if appropriate.

Bob says *'Everyone does the leap according to their capabilities. Using 2 chairs, one on each side, makes it possible for the less mobile of us to have a go.'*

In this context, the posture **Hanumanasana**, usually known as the **Splits** (see page 56), can be considered a bridge between two worlds. The front leg stretches forward into another world while the back leg is a restraining force connecting the body to the earth.

A detailed exposition of the posture can be found in **Anatomy for Hip Openers and Forward Bends** by Ray Long, MD, FRCSC [1].

About twenty years a go I was introduced to the Hunuman's Leap by my teacher Nicolette King. Since then I have been able to piece together two more postures that help to complete the story.

The famous Hanuman's Leap occurred when Hanuman who was King of the Monkeys leapt from India to Ceylon. He did this to rescue the wife of his friend Prince Rama who had been abducted by the Evil Spirit of the Forest.

The Start

Starting from Tadasana take a stride forward and bend the front knee. Then very very quickly raise the arms and come into Warrior 1.

The Hunuman's Pose.

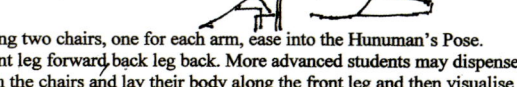

Using two chairs, one for each arm, ease into the Hunuman's Pose. Front leg forward, back leg back. More advanced students may dispense with the chairs and lay their body along the front leg and then visualise that they are flying above the clouds like a rocket.

The Descent.

On arrival over Ceylon ease back into Warrior 1 and very very slowly, palms down, lower the hands, feel as though you are actually pressing against the air, or pressing down through the clouds. Feel the energy in your hands.

Make the return journey using other foot.

Bob Camp
January 2013.

> **The story comes from the Ramayama. After the death of his father, King Dasharatha, Rama is forced to relinquish his right to the throne by going into exile in the forests of India for fourteen years. This was because his father was obliged to follow the wishes of one of his wives so her son could be King.**
> **In the forests Rama, his wife Sita and his brother Lakshmana, find many demons are disturbing and terrifying the sages and renunciates (monks). Rama kills thousands of demons. In revenge Ravana, the powerful demon king of Lanka (now Sri Lanka, formerly Ceylon), abducts the beautiful Sita and takes her to his island.**
> **This is where our sequence begins. Hanuman is a trusted servant of Rama. He leaps to Sri Lanka and finds Sita. He gives her Rama's ring and a message from Rama. Then he leaps back to India. Hanuman's Leap is his leap over the sea to rescue Sita. The story is continued on page 55.**

Preparation Arrange the two chairs on your mat as illustrated. The gap between them needs to be wide enough to allow you to manoeuvre between postures. This will depend upon the width of your shoulders.

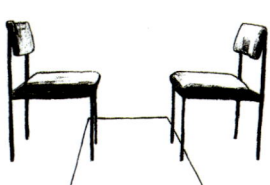
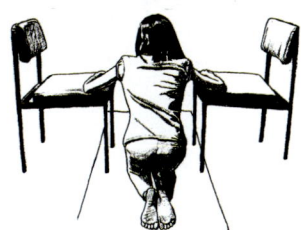

After writing the first draft of this sequence, I was fortunate enough to attend a workshop given by **James Boag** at BWY Congress, 2016. It was titled **Jai Jai Hanuman: Leaping over the Ocean of Samara**.

Afterwards, I asked James if he would edit this sequence and include some of his insights to expand understanding of this inspiring epic. I was confused because I had read so many different interpretations and wanted clarification. Subsequently, I changed some of my text but more of James's comments can be found in the **Additional Notes** on page 56.

1. Published by Bandha Yoga Publications, Plattsburgh, NY. ISBN 13:978-1-60743-942-2

Hanuman's Leap continued

The Story

Hanuman prepares to take the gigantic leap over the water.

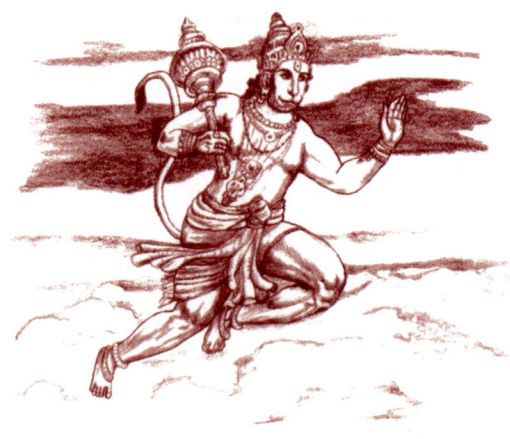

Hanuman takes off and leaps into the air, high above the sea.

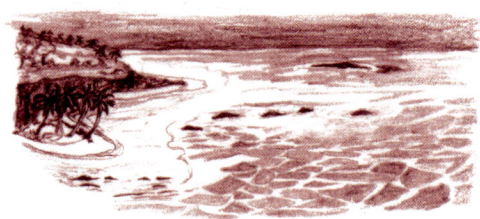

Hanuman moves into the leap towards Sri Lanka.

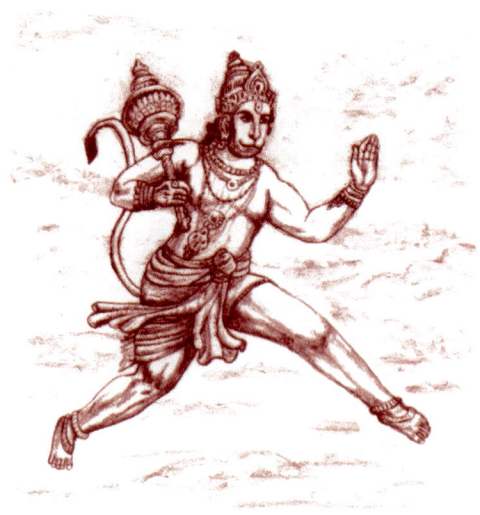

The journey from India to Sri Lanka is about 900 miles (1,500 km). There is a bright blue sky and some white fluffy clouds. The sun is high in the sky. Look down at the sea and imagine you are suspended between two worlds.

The Sequence

1. Stand in front of the chairs with your hands by your sides. Position your self so that when you take a large step forwards, in preparation for **Warrior 1**, your right foot will be in the middle of the gap between the chairs.

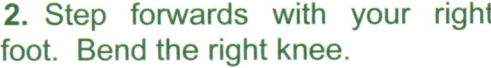

2. Step forwards with your right foot. Bend the right knee.

3. Raise your arms very quickly coming into **Warrior 1**. You can say 'Whoosh' if you like to reinforce the feeling of leaping into the air and taking off.

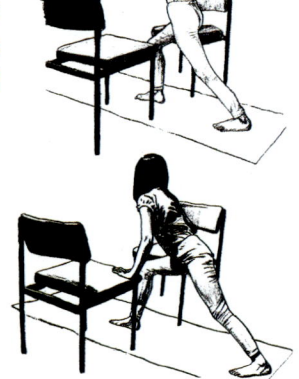

4. Lower your hands to the chair.

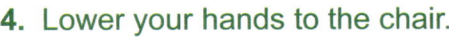

5. Lower your left knee to the floor and place your forearms on the chair as illustrated.

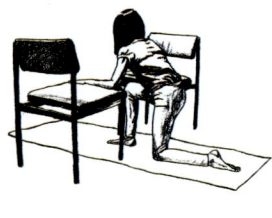

6. Stretch your right leg out in front moving into **Hanumanasana**. While you imagine yourself suspended in the sky, high above the sea, you can experiment with lowering your head and then leaning backwards, as in **7**.

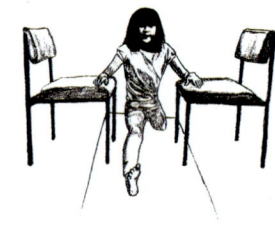

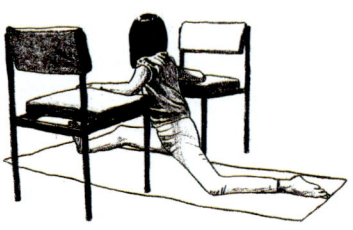

If you feel comfortable in this position, try rotating the back thigh outwards and the heel towards the ceiling. It may help if the back knee is moving slightly to the right.

Hanuman sees the shoreline in the distance and prepares to land.

In the illustration on the opposite page Hanuman is holding a Mace or Gada. In Indian Mythology it is carried by individuals who possess extremely powerful pranic energy (life force).
Although it can be a very dangerous weapon, when associated with gunpowder, for example, when carried by Hanuman, it is more a representation of the power of moral and spiritual integrity.

Hanuman descends slowly, smoothly and gracefully to the island below.

Hanuman lands on the seashore and feels the sand between his toes.

Hanuman searches the city of Lanka (see page 56) until he finds Sita. He gives her Rama's ring and message, comforts her and tells her help is on the way.

7. Slide your right foot back, returning to 5. Move the bent front knee forwards, coming into a Deep Lunge. Feel the stretch at the top of the thighs. Experiment with leaning forwards and backwards, as illustrated.

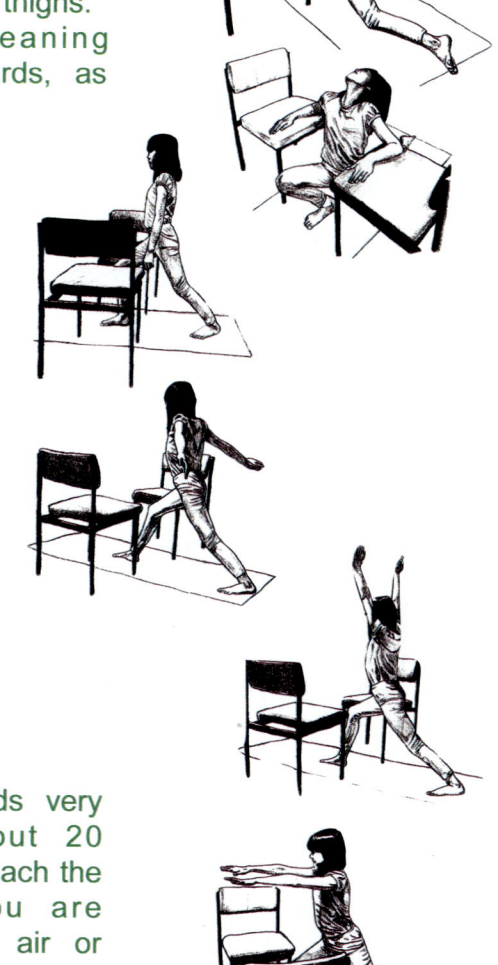

8. Push up on your right foot and hands, returning to **2**.

9. The hands swoop back behind and above your head.

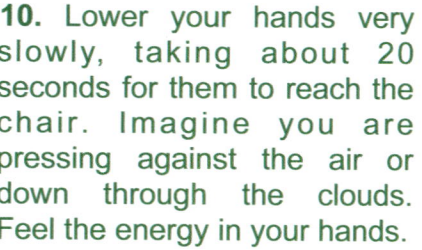

10. Lower your hands very slowly, taking about 20 seconds for them to reach the chair. Imagine you are pressing against the air or down through the clouds. Feel the energy in your hands.

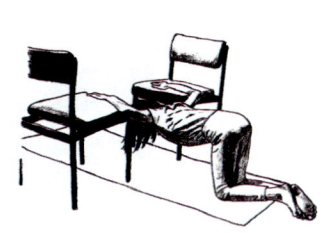

11. Bring your right foot back in front of the chairs. Lower the knees to the floor. Place your forearms on the chairs. Allow your chest to lower and press the shoulder blades together. Keep your head in line with the spine. Pause while you contemplate your adventures.

Mission accomplished, Hanuman prepares for the return journey.

12. **Return to 1.**

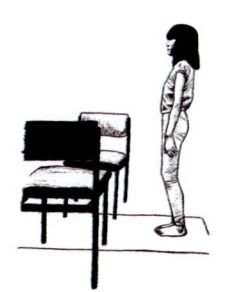

Hanuman leaps back to India.
Change sides and repeat

Variations

You can experiment with going up on the back toes instead of lowering your knee to the floor in **5**, and with your hands on the chair instead of your forearms. You can stay like this from **5** to **8**.

Here are some examples.

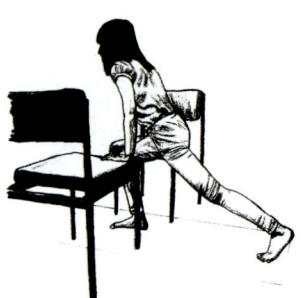

Preparation

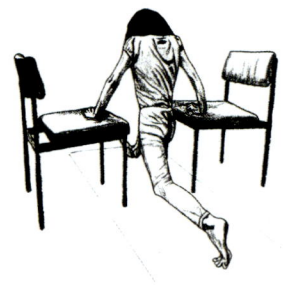

Slide the front foot forwards, as in 6

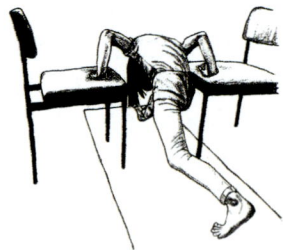

Lean forwards

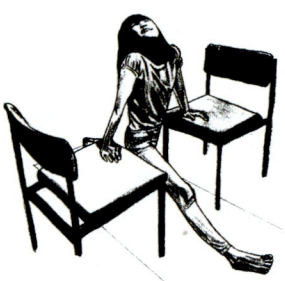

Lean backwards

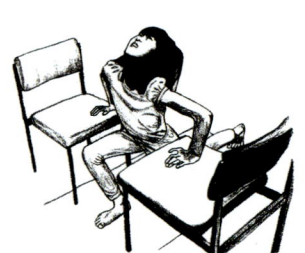

In the Deep Lunge, the elbows can be back or out to the sides

When you come down to land in **10**, you can lift the right leg. Bend the right knee and swing it over to the left, bend the elbows and sink the chest down low. Bring the shoulder blades together and keep the neck in line with the spine.

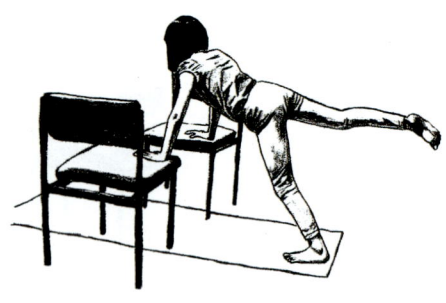

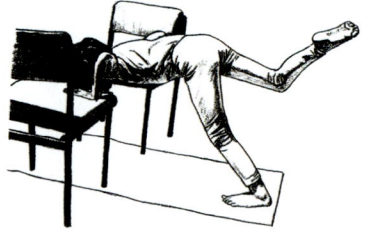

Instead of lowering the knees to the floor in **11**, you can move the hips backwards. The knees can be straight or bent. Broaden the shoulders and sink the chest down.

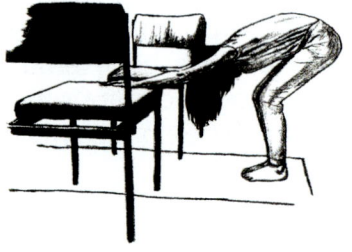

It was the greatest leap ever taken. The speed of Hanuman's jump pulled blossoms and flowers into the air after him and they fell like little stars on the waving treetops. The animals on the beach had never seen such a thing; they cheered Hanuman, then the air burned from his passage, and red clouds flamed over the sky… (Ramayana, retold by William Buck).

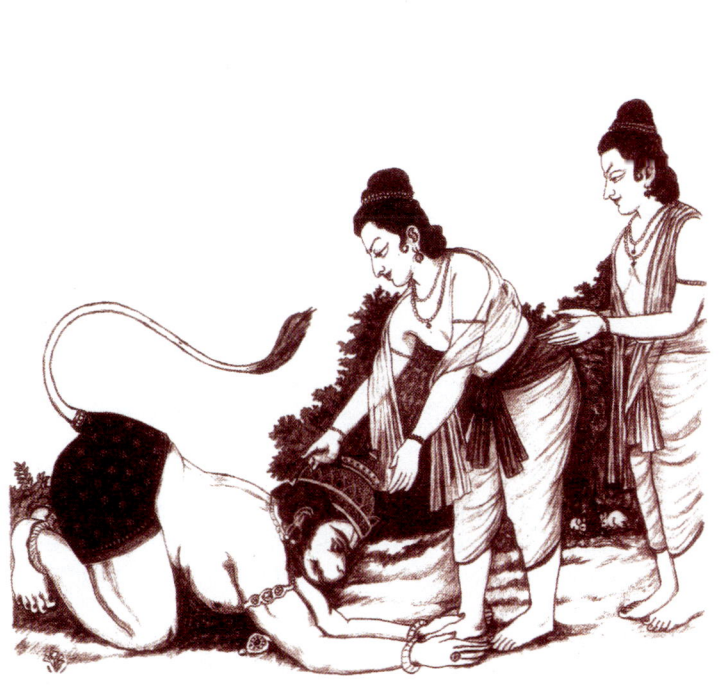

Hanuman greets Rama and Lakshmana in the forest

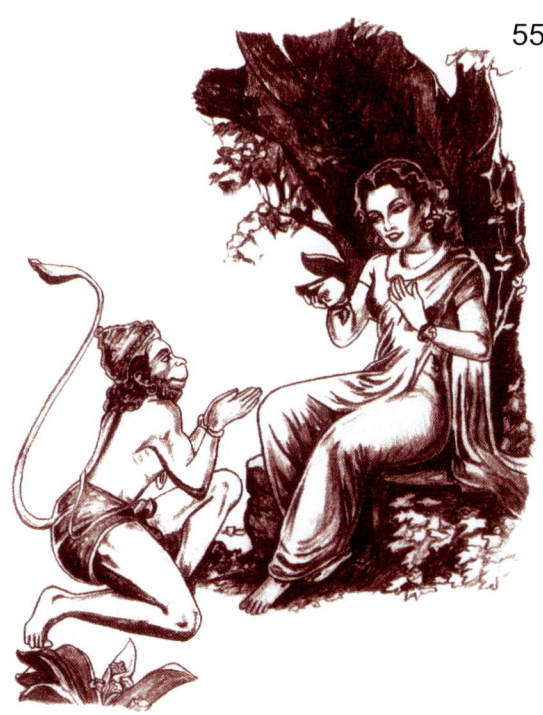

Hanuman finds Sita and gives her Rama's ring and message

The story continued:

Hanuman tells Rama where Sita is being held captive.

The monkeys build a bridge from India to the island and Rama's army and the monkey warriors cross over to Lanka.

Eventually all the armies meet and the Battle of Lanka ensues.

Ravana has 10 heads. Rama slays Ravana and the demons are destroyed. This is a triumph of **good** over **evil**. Rama rescues Sita and peace is restored in the world.

Observations

I came across different interpretations of Hanuman and his story while researching background information for this sequence. To some of his many devotees he is a partial incarnation of Lord Siva (The destroyer of things past their use by date. This makes way for the renewal process). Sometimes Rama is called Ram.

However, it became obvious that the character of Hanuman has captured the imagination of many hearts. I became quite intrigued by him and have even involved him in my meditations, see page 105.

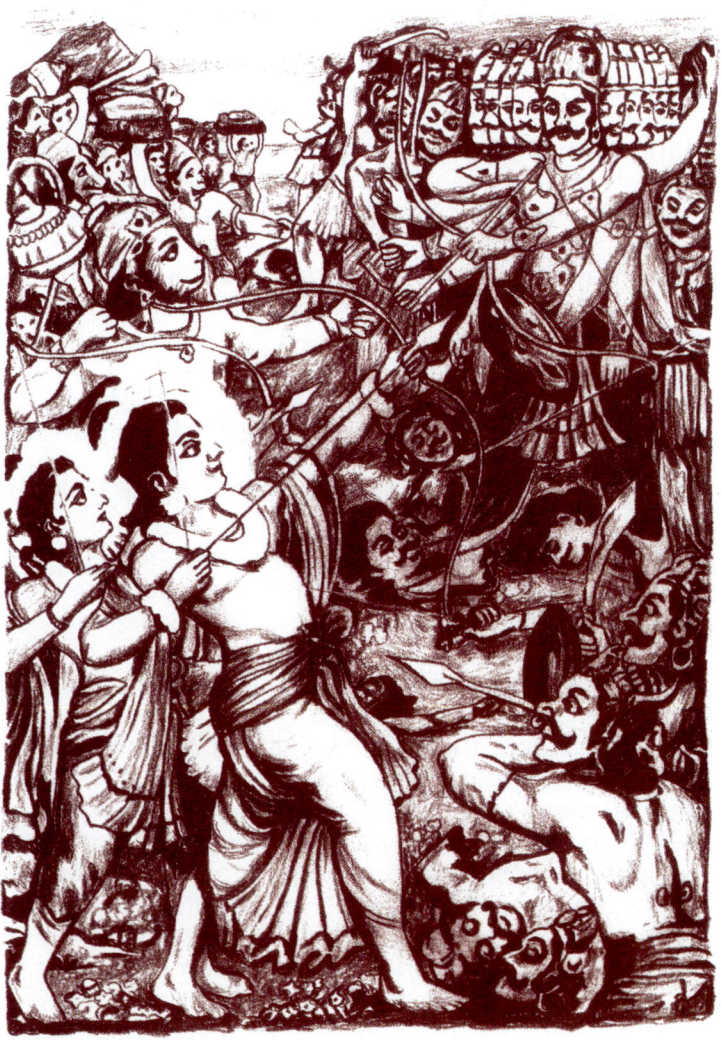

The Battle of Lanka

Additional Notes

The Splits?

Sometimes **Hanumanasana** is called the **Splits**, but in this context, that is a bit misleading. Even though one leg reaches forwards and the other to the rear, they both connect back to and feed into the centre. The posture is about **balance** and **integration**, not splitting apart! Hanuman is the opposite of a 'split personality'. He is a **Siddha**, a master yogin, who has integrated all his incarnate powers and gifts in service of his beloved Rama.

The posture known as **Hanumanasana**, can be considered a bridge between two worlds, or **planes of understanding**. The **front leg** stretches forwards into another world, into **the unknown**, while the **back leg** is a restraining force connecting the body to **the earth** and keeping us connected to our grounding wisdom.

The Ramayana is one of two great epics (along with Mahabharata) of the Indian Tradition. It is the first great Epic Poem[1] in the Sanskrit[2] tradition, **and conveys**, through the riveting, beautiful and sometimes troublingly thought-provoking story of Prince **Rama**, the teachings of yoga.

Scholars hold a range of opinions about when the Ramayana was authored, but agree that it dates back, at the very least, to the so called 'Epic Age 'of Indian Literature, ca.600BC – 100BC.

Rama is considered an incarnation or avatar of **Vishnu, the preserver of the material world**. He was destined to overcome forces of tyranny and fearful fragmentation and re-establish **dharma, balance and harmony through the realms of existence**. He is held up in the orthodox Indian tradition as the example or embodiment of a **perfect human being** and is respected as a good, compassionate King. He lived in the Vedic era, between about 3,000 and 2,500 BC.

Hanuman is one of the great heroes of the epic Ramayana and one of the most popular aspects or representations of the **divine** in the Indian tradition. He is one of the great **vanaras**, forest dwelling beings with monkey-like head and tail, who help Rama to rescue Sita.

Hanuman is considered a partial incarnation of **Siva**, and is known as **the son of the wind**, because the wind was instrumental in delivering the seed with which his mother **Anjani** conceived him.

He is sometimes called 'King of the Monkeys' but this is not accurate. He is a great minister to **Sugriva**, the **exiled King of the Vanaras** (see above, forest dwelling beings).

Symbolically and archetypically, it is important that Hanuman is a minister, messenger, servant and warrior, but not a King. It is his completion of each of these roles that allows Rama to become King. In other words, as an individual soul uses his/her conscious gifts in service of the soul's deepest longings, then the soul can become established on the seat/throne of enlightenment.

The city? I wrote 'forest' but James explained that **Sita** was found in a city.

In Ramayana, Lanka is a citadel island. The majestic city was designed and fashioned by **Vishwakarman**, the celestial architect, for **Kubera**, god of wealth and riches. **Kubera** had it as his base until mighty **Ravana** kicked him out and took it, as the most splendid palace available, for his own. It is an island kingdom, with a central palace, surrounded by an amazing walled city. **Hanuman** marvels at the sophistication, beauty and opulence of the walled city and **Ravana's** amazing palace. He searches for **Sita** high and low through the city and its parks and neighbourhoods to a point of despair. Only the way the sunlight falls alerts him to a place he has not yet searched, and he then finds **Sita** deep within **Ravana's** magnificent palace in a walled secret garden that encloses a beautiful forest grove. This is why **Hanuman** and **Sita** are depicted in a forested setting. It is a slice of the forest in the middle of the city.

Symbolically, as **Ravana's** very well-constructed palace and citadel surrounded by the great moat of the ocean can be seen to represent the constructs and well-established, familiar patterns of the minds, and the limits of our conditioning, the forest grove, with **Sita** in it, can be seen as the wild heart that can never be tamed, the deep intuitive wisdom of the spirit that can be shrouded and repressed, but never extinguished.

James Boag is a Sanskrit scholar and teaches applied yoga philosophy and mythology around the world. Drawing on his background in languages and scriptural teaching, he brings the practical essence of traditional Indian teachings into the vivid context of our human lives today. www.jamesboagyoga.com

An animated film of the Ramayana, '**The Legend of Prince Rama**' was made in Japan in 1992 by Yugo Sako. It can be watched on YouTube at www.youtube.com/watch?v=JSB1wKHT_hy.

1. An Epic is a long narrative poem that records heroic events in an elevated style.
2. Sanskrit is an ancient Indian language of Hinduism and the Vedas and is the classical literary language of India.

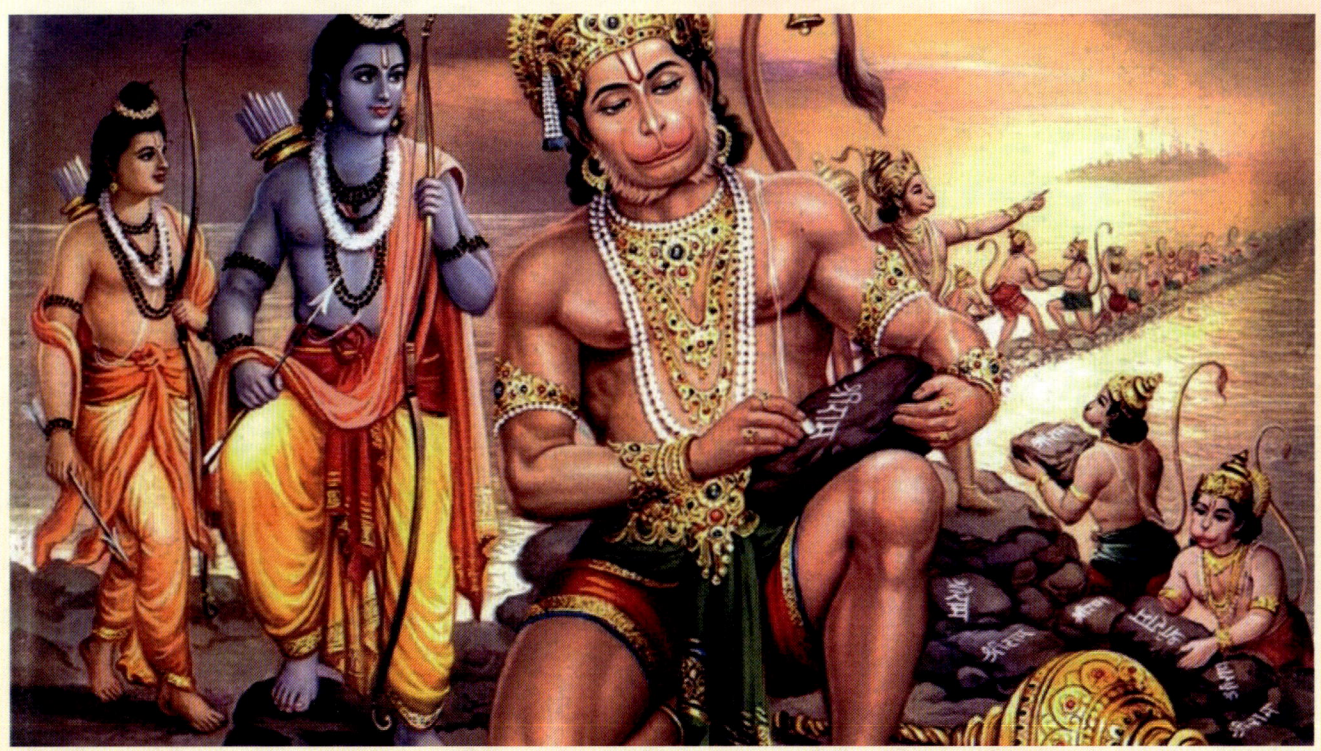

Hanuman, Ram and Lakshmana and the monkeys building the bridge between India and the island of Lanka

Painting from a Google, Free Image site. The artists name was not included.

Gate Variations

This sequence repeats the same three postures with their variations. There is a different posture linking them together each time they are repeated.

Hold each posture for at least three breaths and increase the stretches on the exhalations.

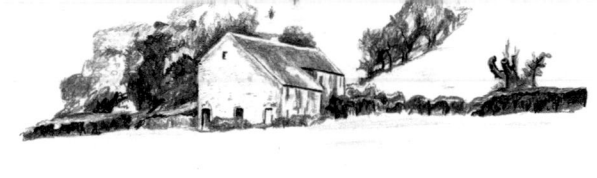

1. Kneel on the right knee and straighten your left leg out to the side. Bring your hands into **Prayer**.

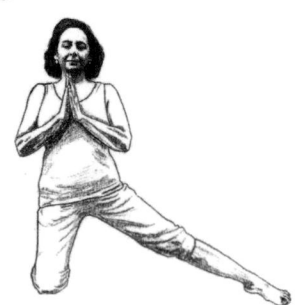

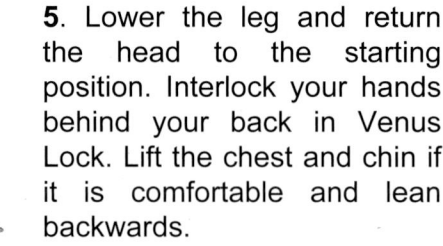

5. Lower the leg and return the head to the starting position. Interlock your hands behind your back in Venus Lock. Lift the chest and chin if it is comfortable and lean backwards.

2. Place your left hand on the left knee and bring the right hand up over your head. Gradually increase the stretch to the left in the **Gate** posture. The left hand slides further down your leg.

6. Return to **2**, but this time, catch hold of your right wrist with your left hand and pull yourself over to the left.

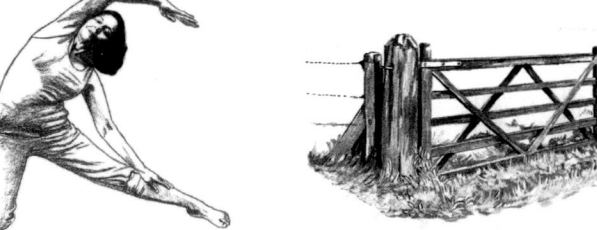

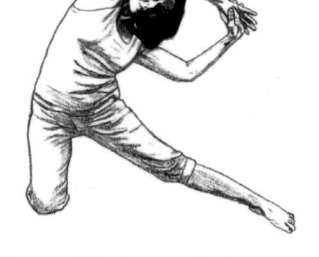

3. Lower your right hand to the floor and stretch your left hand over your head. Enjoy the stretch along the left side of your body from the fingers to the toes. Keep the left shoulder back and look up.

7. Return to 3 and then lift the left leg a short distance off the floor. Continue to stretch fingers away from toes on the **exhalations**.

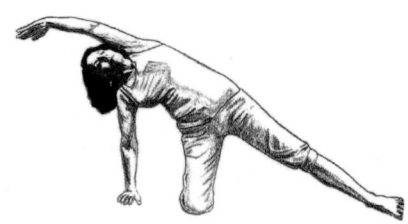

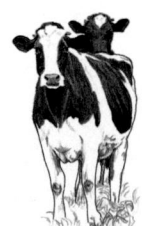

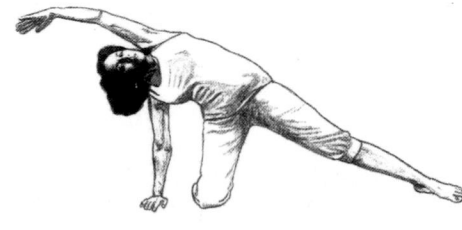

4. Lift your left leg and stretch your left hand up to the ceiling

8. Lift the left leg and place the hand on your hip. Bring your left shoulder back rotating the chest as far round as it will go and look up.

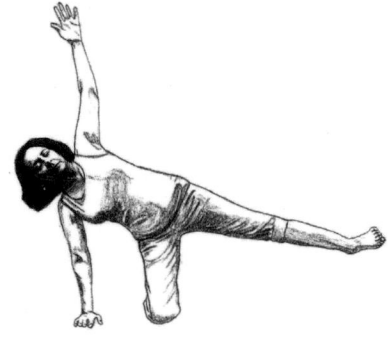

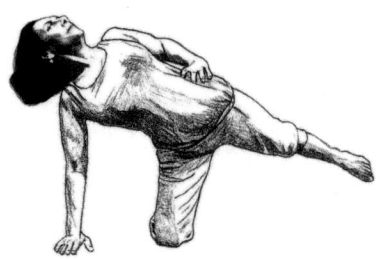

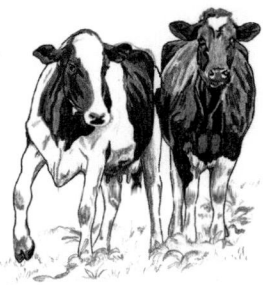

9. Lower the leg but keep your hand on the hip. Rotate to the right and place the right hand on your heel.

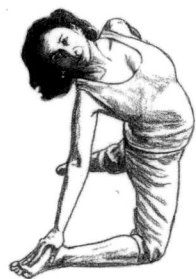

10. Return to **2** but with the right hand on your head. Bring the right shoulder back and look up. Continue as before.

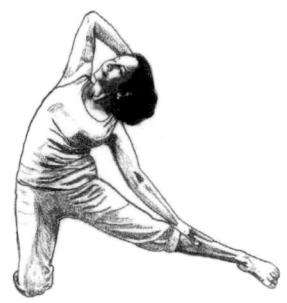

11. Return to **7**. This time you are going to swing your leg backwards and forwards in the **Swinging Gate**. After a few repetitions, pause in the backward position and experience the interesting curve of your body.

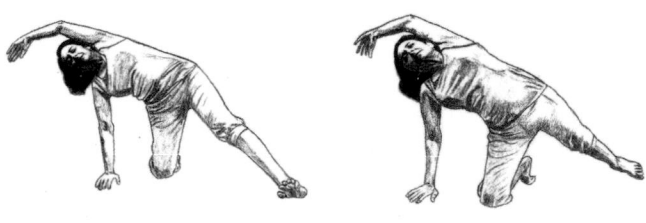

12. Return to **8** but this time slide the left hand behind your back as far as it will go and rotate round even more.

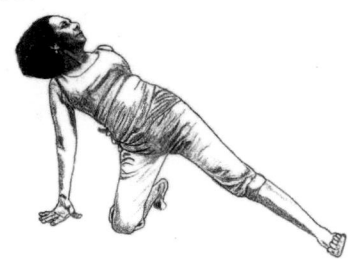

13. Lower the leg and replace your hand on your head. Rotate over the left leg and lower the head towards the knee.

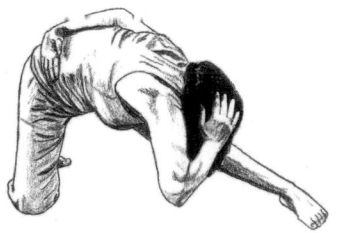

14. Return to **2** but with the back of your hand on your knee and lift your toes so that your weight is on the heel.

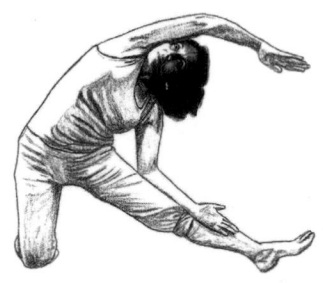

15. When you feel you can't stretch anymore to the left, lower your toes to the floor. Move even further into the stretch, sliding the back of your hand lower down the leg.

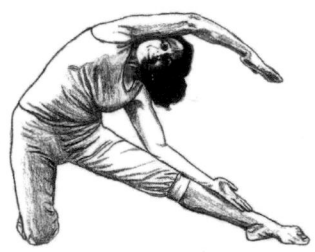

16. Repeat 3 and 4, increasing the stretches even more the second time around, before returning to 1.

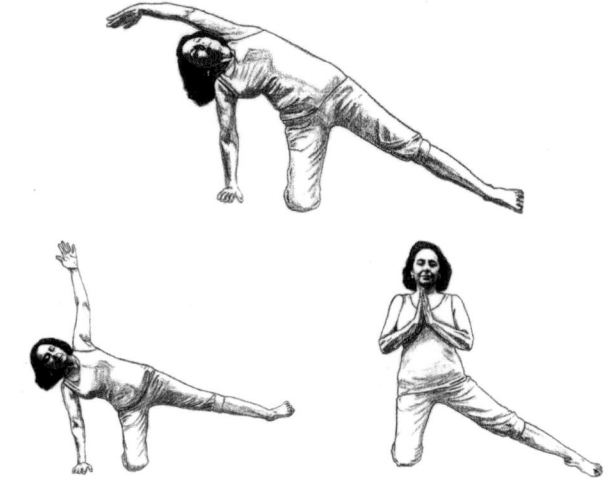

Change sides and repeat

Seated Gate Variations

This is a simplified version of the **Gate Variations** as demonstrated by my 95-year-old pupil.
The same suggestions apply:

Hold each posture for at least three breaths and increase the stretches on the exhalations.

It is necessary to sit at the front of the chair. The seat must not be too high. You need to be able to place one foot firmly on the floor with the knee bent.
You may rest the backward shoulder on the back of the chair in some of the postures if it feels comfortable, e.g., **2**, **3** and **6**.

1. With the right knee bent and the left leg straight, place your left hand on the knee. Curve the right arm over your head and stretch over to the left.

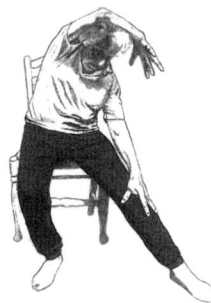

2. Find a convenient part at the sides or back of the chair for your right hand to hold on to.
Bring your left hand over your head and stretch the fingers away from your toes. Enjoy the stretch along the left side.

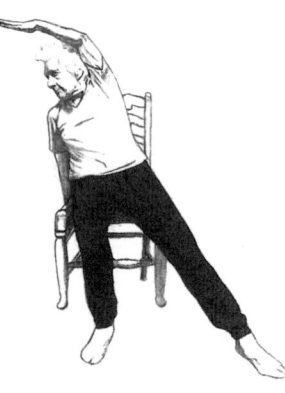

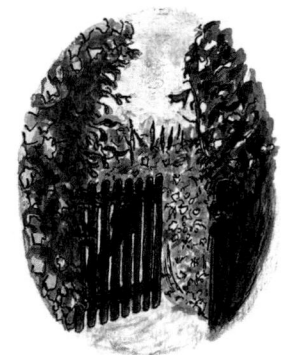

3. Lift your left hand and foot and stretch away.

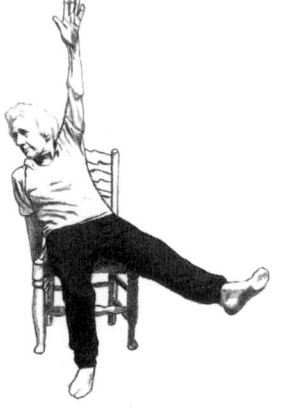

4. Lower the hand and foot. Curve the right hand over your head and catch hold of the wrist with your left hand and pull the upper body over to the left.

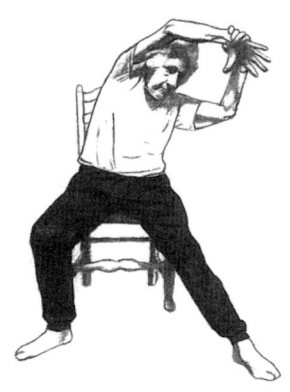

5. Return to **2** and lift the left foot a short distance off the floor.

6. Place the left hand on your hip and lift the left leg. Twist round to the right but move your left shoulder backwards, opening out the chest.

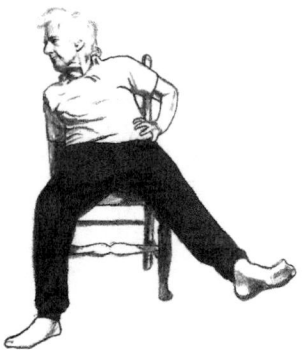

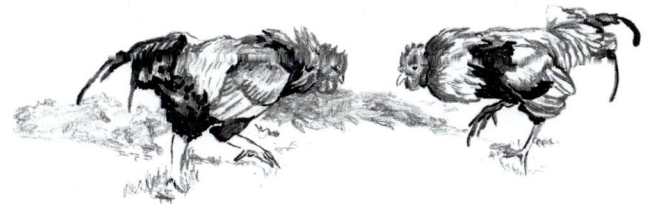

10. Lower the leg and place the back of the left hand on your knee. Curve the right arm over your head and go up on your left heel, lifting your toes.

Slowly slide the back of your hand down your leg as you increase the stretch to the left. Keep the right shoulder back.

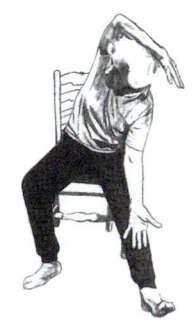

7. Lower the leg and place the right hand on your head and left hand on your knee. Keep your right shoulder back and look up to the right as you gradually lower to the left.

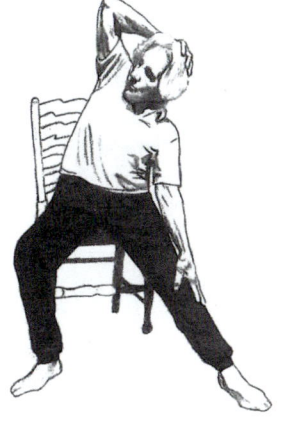

8. Return to **5**.

11. When you have stretched as far as you can, lower the toes to the floor and then slide your hand a little further down your leg until you find your maximum stretch in this pose.

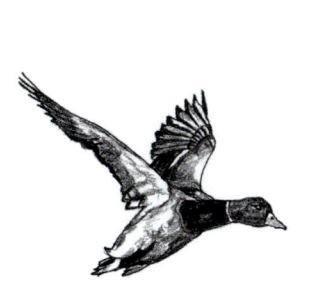

To conclude, repeat **2** and **3** and *change sides and repeat.*

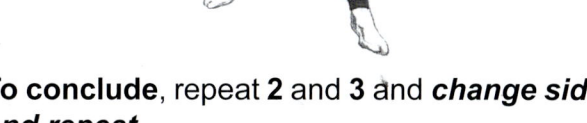

9. Lower the left hand and slide it round behind your back. Lift the left leg and twist round to the right as in **6**.

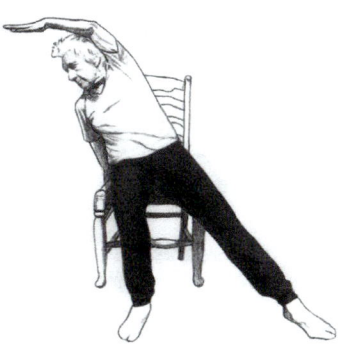

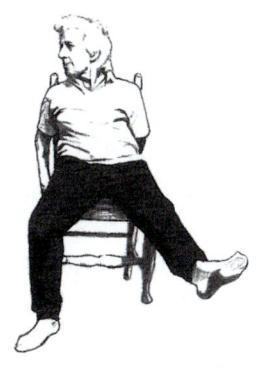

These are the basic versions of the postures but you can make them more strenuous. In **5**, **6** and **9** you can slide your right arm down the back leg of the chair and you can hold the postures for much longer.

Some people like to sit on a front corner of the chair. You may have to adapt the sequence to accommodate the chairs you are using.

Twisting and Sliding Sequence

I met up with Tasha, a dynamic young yoga teacher from 'Tranquillity in the City', to exchange ideas. Some of her innovations were floor twists. I wanted to use them but they took up a lot of floor space, so I modified them, put them all together in a **sliding down your mat** sequence and added a few more.

The standing postures at the beginning and end are inspired by Dru Yoga. They seemed to compliment the postures on the mat.

1. Stand with the feet together or a hip-width apart or wider. This is an idea you can experiment with and repeat as many times as you want to. If you have problematic knees, you may prefer to stand with the feet together.

Choose a slow and steady pace and maintain it throughout.

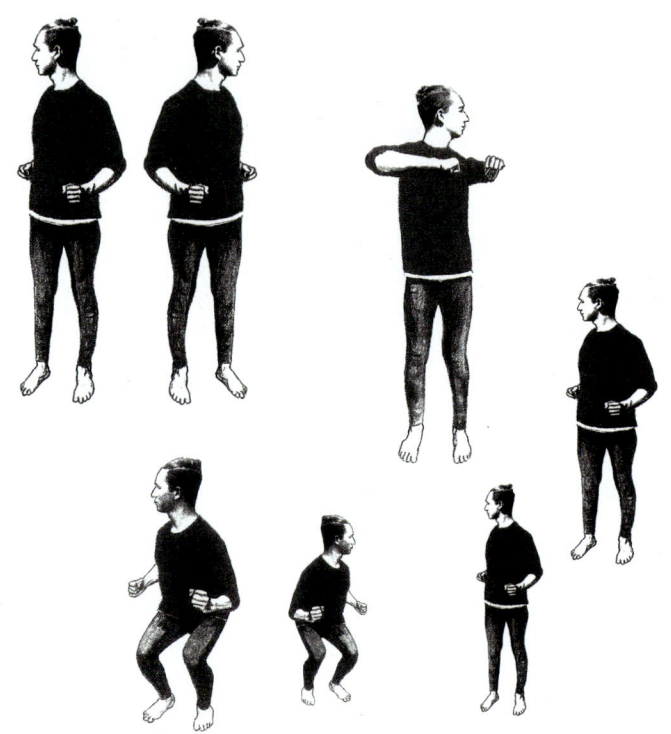

A. Clench your fists with the palms facing. With your arms at your sides, bend your elbows. Start to twist round from side to side. The emphasis will be on twisting from the waist.

B. Gradually move your awareness up your body to the shoulders and lift the elbows up to shoulder level.

C. Move your awareness back to the waist and lower the elbows.

D. Gradually bend your knees and squat down. The elbows will follow you down.

E. When you are ready, twist back to the starting point.

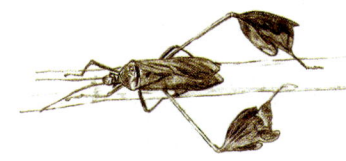

A Stick Insect manoeuvres its way along a branch.

2. We are aiming to manoeuvre ourselves from one end of the mat to the other. If you are a small child, you may not reach the end of the mat. That doesn't matter. If you are very tall, you may need two mat lengths. For practical reasons, choose to do each set of movements a certain number of times. I suggest eight times - four times each side. You can vary this but keep the number you choose consistent.

The first time you try this mat work you may not enjoy it or feel it is worth the effort, but it improves with practise. You may need to experiment with it before you feel the benefits.

No breathing suggestions are given in this section. Observe the breathing pattern your body adopts in the repetitions. It will be interesting to compare notes afterwards.

Sometimes non-slip mats can be counterproductive, e.g., when you try to slide your heel forwards in **Hanumanasana** and you can't. You may find some resistance from your mat as you try to slide along it and need to summon up some extra energy to compensate for that. If you are practising at home, you could try on a carpet without using a mat, making the suggested eight movements per section.

A. Lie on your back with your head at the top of the mat. Bend your knees with the feet together and place your hands to the sides with the palms facing downwards.

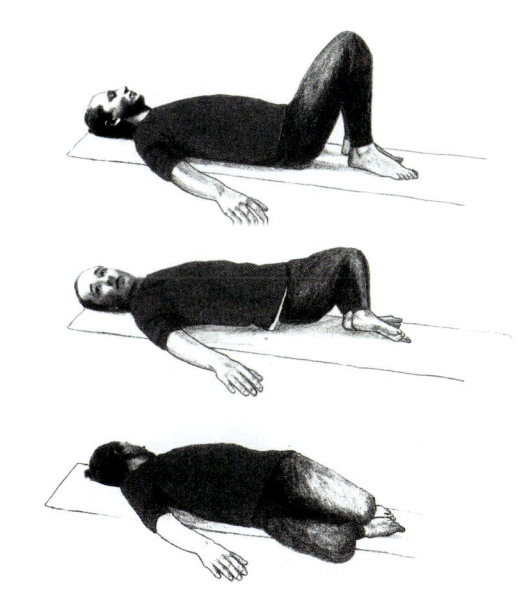

B. Look to the right and swing your knees to the left. This is usually called **Windscreen Wipers**.

C. Change sides and, as you swing your knees and head in the other direction, slide a little further down the mat.

Continue to twist from side to side, manoeuvring slowly down the mat another six times or for your chosen number of times.

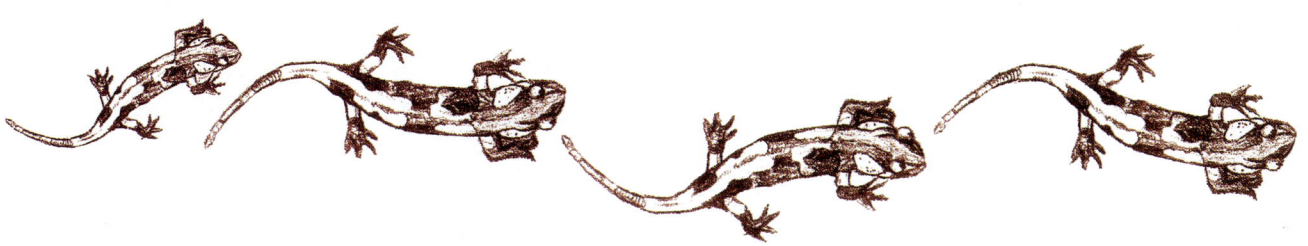

3. To reposition yourself, move to a sitting posture with the hands behind. Lift the feet with the soles together and the knees out to the sides. Shuffle round in a semi-circle in either direction until you are facing in the opposite direction.

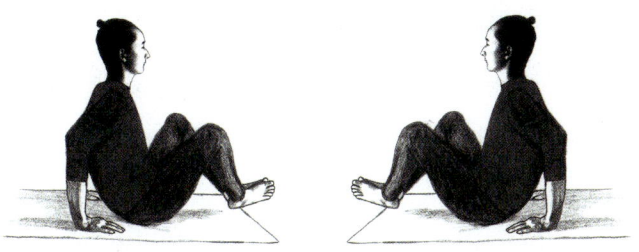

4A. Lie on your back with your left leg straight and your right knee bent.
Look to the right and swing your right knee to the left. Aim to touch the floor with your big toe. The hips will come off the floor. Some people will be able to keep both shoulders on the floor, others will need to lift the right one. Either way, encourage the right shoulder away from the right knee.

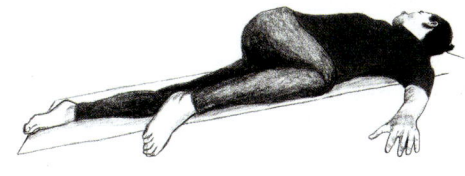

B. As you swing your right leg back, straighten it and stretch it forwards. At the same time, bend your left knee. This is when you adjust your position on the mat.
Repeat as above, swinging your left knee over to the right and looking to the left.
Continue to twist and slide down your mat.

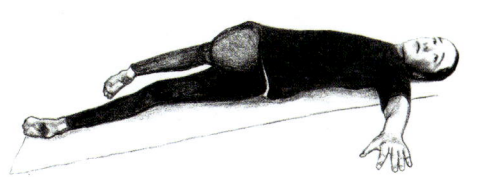

5. Roll over onto your front. We are going to repeat these twists face downwards. You can choose to use your arms in different ways to accommodate your body type.

You can start with your hands together, either with one on top of the other as in **7A**, or with the fingers facing each other. You can slide the elbows forwards and backwards to help the sliding process.

You can place your hands at the edge of the mat with the fingers turned inwards. The chest can be low or high as in **5A** and **B**.

5A and **B**. Repeat as in **2A** and **B,** only this time you will be face downwards.

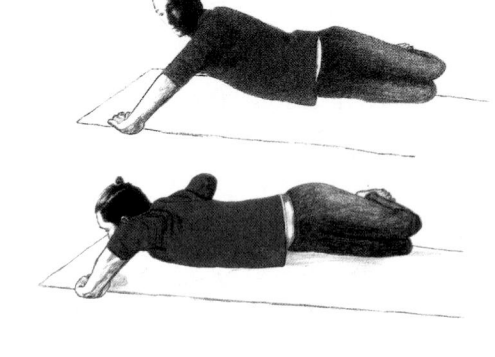

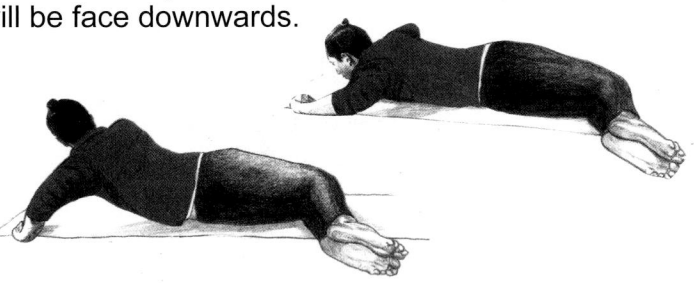

6. When you get to the end of the mat, bend your knees and bring your hands further back. Slowly manoeuvre yourself in a semi circle so that you are facing in the other direction.

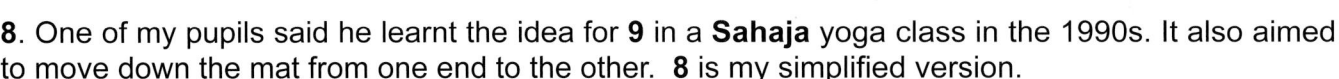

7. **A** and **B**. Choose the position of your hands and repeat **4 A** and **B** on your front.

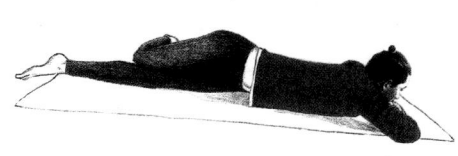

8. One of my pupils said he learnt the idea for **9** in a **Sahaja** yoga class in the 1990s. It also aimed to move down the mat from one end to the other. **8** is my simplified version.

A. Sit at the end of your mat with the hands on the floor behind and the fingers turned backwards. Bend the knees and place the feet on the edge of your mat.

B. Let the right knee fall out to the side and lower your left knee to the sole of your right foot.

C. Return to **A**.

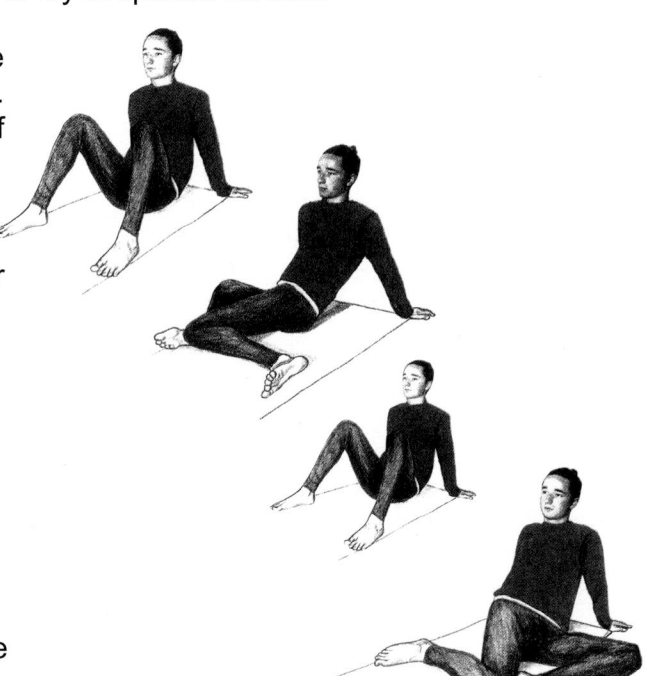

D. Change sides and repeat. With each twist, move a little down the mat.

9A. Start as in **8A** but with your hands above your head.

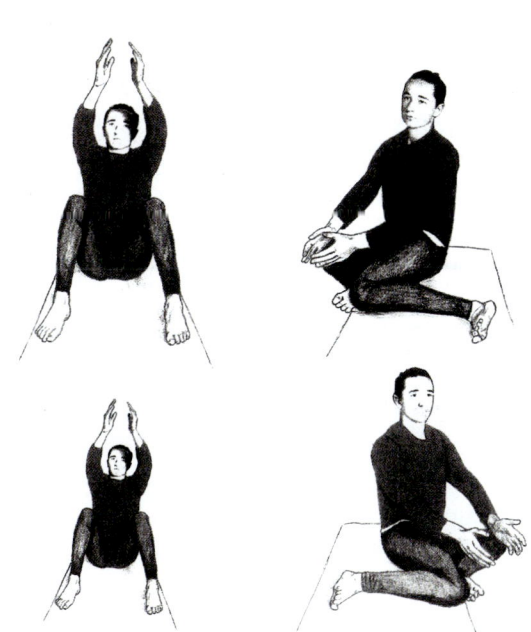

B. As you lower your knees to the right, lower your hands in the same direction.

C. Return to **A** and change sides. Continue for your chosen duration.

10A. Start at one end of your mat face downwards with the right forearm across the mat, as illustrated. Stretch your left arm forwards and swing your left leg over to the right. Both can be at a 45 degree angle away from the body so that they can be stretched away from each other in a straight line.

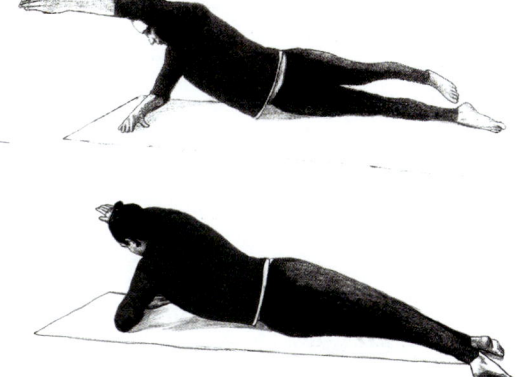

B. Each time you change sides, place the opposite forearm behind the other one so that you are slowly moving down the mat.

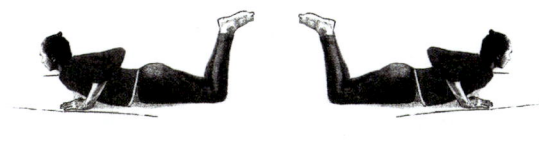

11. When you get to the end of the mat, manoeuvre yourself round as suggested in **6**.

12 A. Place your right forearm across the mat and roll over onto your right side. With the left foot on top of the right foot, raise your left hand and lift the hips.

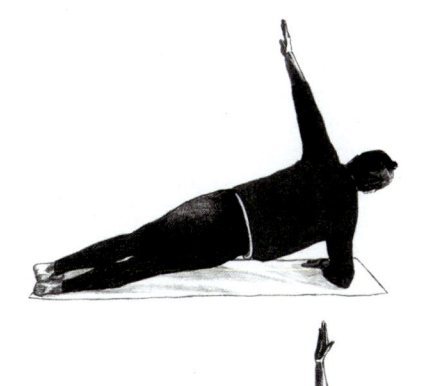

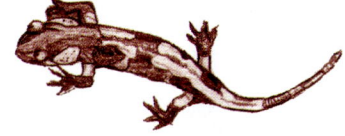

B. Change sides as above, in **10B**, placing the left forearm behind the right one. Proceed in the same way.

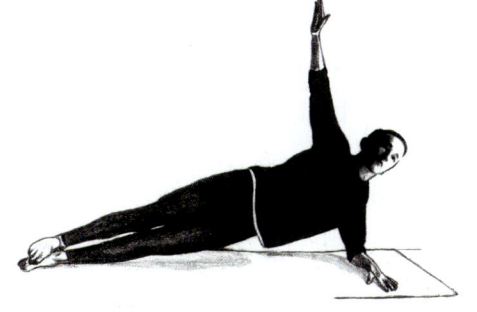

13. This practice is from a **Dru Yoga** video by **Annie Jones**. She calls it a **Liver Detox**. It repeatedly twists the area above the waist.

A. Stand with the feet a hip-width apart and the arms parallel to the floor. Push away with the palms of your hands.

B. INHALE as you turn your right palm upwards and bring your right elbow back, twisting round to the right. The head follows the twist. Push away with your left hand.

C. EXHALE back to **A**.

D. INHALE as you twist round to the left, repeating the procedure.

E. EXHALE back to **A**.

The drawing above is of a South American Tree Frog.

F. After repeating this a few times, twist round to one side on the **inhalation** and round to the other side on the **exhalation**.
After about eight breaths, switch sides and continue for the same number of breaths.

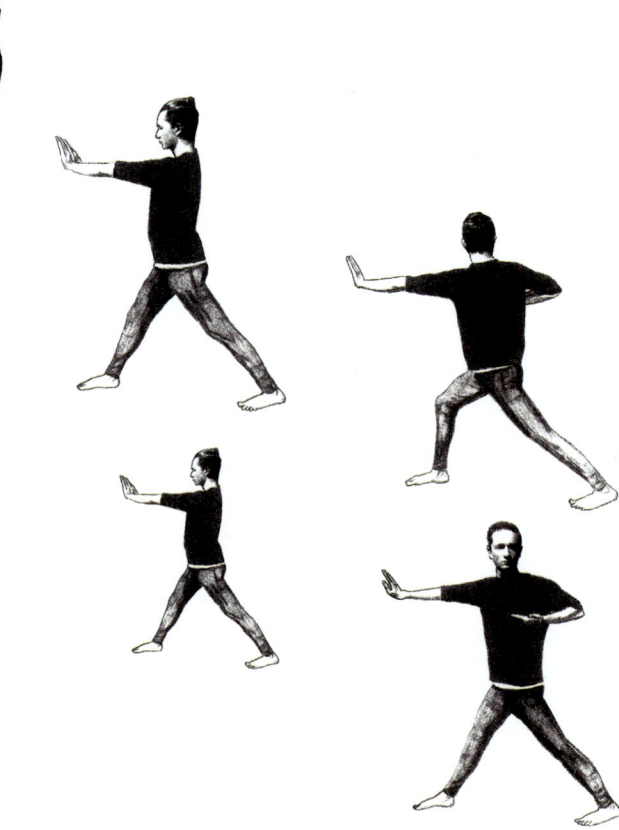

G. From the same starting position, **13A**, step forwards with the right foot.

H. Bend the right knee as you **INHALE** and bring your right elbow back with the palm facing upwards, as in **13B**.
You can lift the back heel off the floor as you bend the right knee if it feels comfortable.

I. EXHALE back to **G**.

J. Straighten the right leg as you **EXHALE** and twist round to the left, reversing sides.

After repeating this a few times, adapt the instructions in **F** to this variation.

More variations

After I finished setting out this sequence the ideas kept coming. Here are some more to mix and match with the previous pages.

1. Start as in **2A** then place your right foot over the left knee.

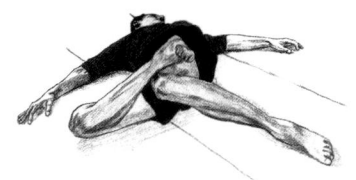

2. Lower the right knee to the floor and look to the left.

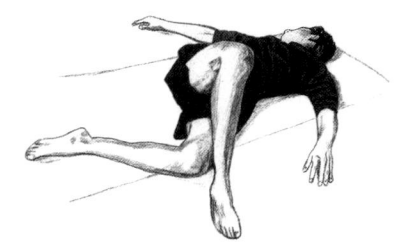

3. Swing the legs over to the other side. Try to place the whole of the sole of your foot on the floor and look to the right. *Continue as before, manoeuvring down the mat for your chosen number of twists.*

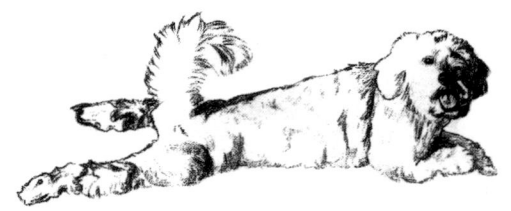

This is Yoyo, one of my pupils' dogs. She enjoys sliding along the floor, paddling with her front legs while her back legs remain passive.

One of my pupils suggested this variation. You can use it instead of **3** on page 63 so that you return to the top end of your mat.

1. When you find yourself at the bottom end of your mat, you can slide yourself back to the starting point.
Bring the left foot back as far as it will go. Push on it to manoeuvre up the mat. As you do this, curve your trunk and head to the right.

2. Repeat bringing your right foot back and curving your body to the left. *Continue until you are back where you started*.

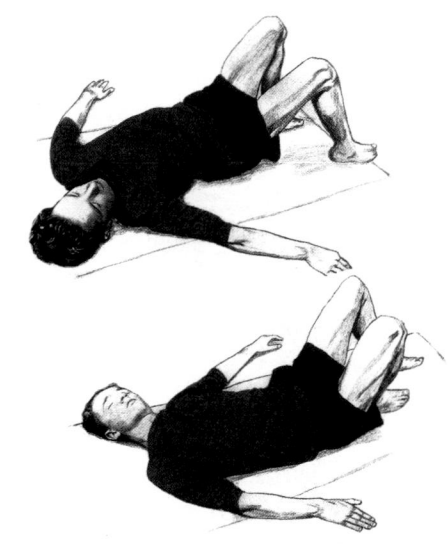

More variations continued

I attended a class given by **Dr Hania Katarina Kramlund** at the beautiful **Mandala Yoga Ashram** in South Wales. She included these supine twists which she called the **Cork Screw**. She didn't suggest sliding down the mat or any breathing pattern. My suggestions are in italics.

1. Lie on your back with the legs straight, the feet close together and the arms out wide.

Lower your feet to the right and look to the left. *Try to get the outside of the lower foot to touch the floor.*
Change sides (swing the feet over to the left and look to the right) **and repeat as many times as you want to**.

2. Cross the feet over and proceed as in **1**. *Try to get one of your big toes to the floor each time.*
When you are ready, cross your feet over the other way and repeat.

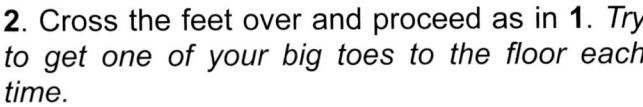

3. Place a heel in between the big toes and second toe.
Repeat as above and then change sides.

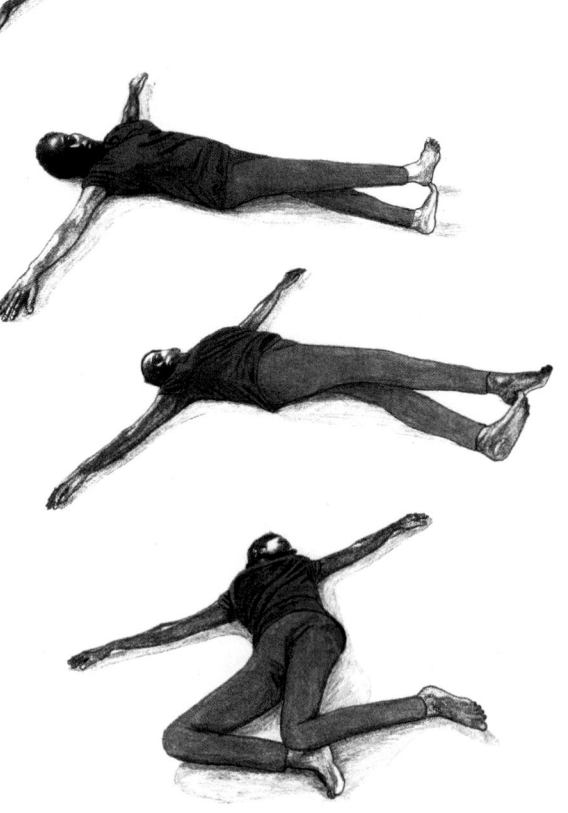

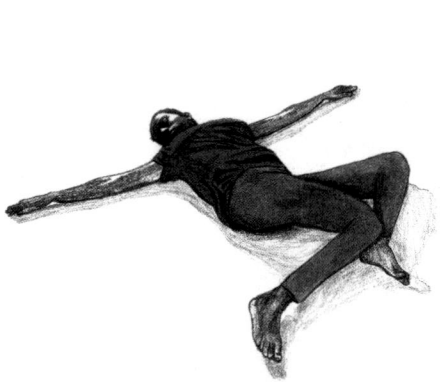

4. **Wide Windscreen Wipers**. Lie on your back with the feet a mat-width apart. Swing your knees slowly from side to side, turning your head in the opposite direction.
Repeat as above.

Caution
If you have a bad neck, it is not necessary to move your head in the opposite direction to your feet. You will still find the sequence beneficial if you keep your head in a neutral position.

I sent Dr. Kramlund my first draft of her sequence and she added two more twists.

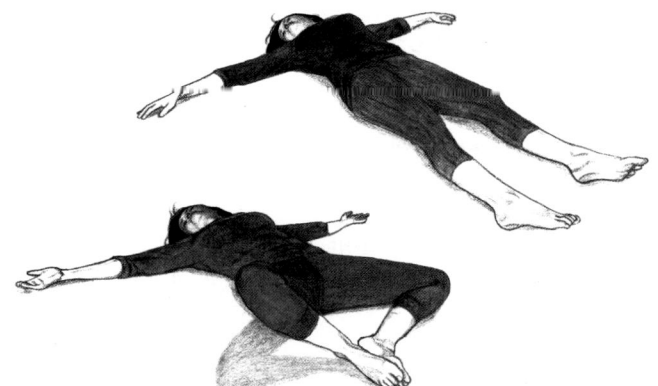

A is the same as **1** but the feet are further apart. You can add this after **1**.

B fits in well at the end of the sequence. The knees lower from side to side as illustrated. The opposite hip can come off the floor. Keep the knees wide apart.

Teachers may find this short sequence useful when they find they have five minutes left at the end of the posture work, before the Final Relaxation.

The Introduction to the Floor and Wall Sequence

This is my final contribution for this book. There were postures I wanted to include and they all involved the floor or wall so I put them all together and hope they make a balanced combination.

The Sources of the Postures
1 to **3** come from old yoga magazines.
4 to **8** are inspired by Dru Yoga.
9 to **11** come from old yoga magazines.
12 to **14** are my own ideas.
15 & **16** are from general yogic repertoire. Paul Grilley calls this **Shoelace on the Wall** in his book **Yin Yoga, Principles and Practice**[1]. He suggests holding the pose for between 3 and 5 minutes to create a stretch in the buttock or thigh.
20 to **23** are inspired by Bruce Bowditch from his book **The Yoga Practice, Guide 2**[2]. He does these postures freestanding and also includes a twist. While in **22**, you could bring an elbow to the supporting thigh.
24 is from general yogic repertoire.
25 comes from a book by Swami Pragyamurti Saraswati called **Yoga Manual for Prisoners and other Castaways**[3]. Swamiji says it is a comfortable pose for pregnant women and it can alleviate sciatic pain.

Cautions
Do not turn your head in the inverted postures, **12** to **19**.
In the postures where you have your back on the wall, **20** to **23**, make sure that your feet can't slip forwards. Stand on a non-slip mat.

Additional notes
As some of my pupils have large tummies, I suggest that they practise **Sitting Forward Bends** with their legs wide apart. This creates space for their tummies and makes the posture more comfortable. **4** and **5** are from the original Dru Yoga concept. You can add holding the heels or legs with the toes pointed, as in **7** and **8**, after **5**.

You can vary postures **9** to **11**, by sitting on one or two blocks quite close to the wall. You can have one knee on top of the other to the side and the feet away from the wall.

Some yoga teachers would suggest placing a folded blanket under the shoulders in postures **12** to **19**. This would be to make the neck less compressed. Some people may find this more comfortable.

1. **Yin Yoga, Principles and Practice** (2002) published by White Cloud Press.
2. **The Yoga Practice, Guide 2** (2012) published by Third Eye Press.
3. **Yoga Manual for Prisoners and other Castaways** (2010) published by SevaUnite Trust.

Floor and Wall Sequence

Sitting postures with the toes pointed.

1. Sit with the legs wide apart and the toes pointed. Place the back of your right hand on the top of your right leg or foot. The elbow can rest on the knee.
INHALE as you lift the left arm. Rotate the shoulder and torso to the left and look up at your hand.

2. **EXHALE** as you bend over to the right. The left arm follows. Hold for a few breaths as you deepen the stretch. Slide the back of your right hand along the top of the leg or foot. Keep looking up to the left and rotating the left shoulder backwards.

3. When you are ready, catch hold of the inside of the heel or inner leg with the palm of the right hand. Place your left hand on the left hip. Keep the head and shoulders low as you twist round to the left.
Hold for a few breaths as you increase the twist. Change sides and repeat.

4. Sit with the feet together, the toes pointed and the hands at heart level with the palms facing upwards. **INHALE**.

5. **EXHALE** as you stretch the hands forwards, as far as you can, without touching the feet. **INHALE** back to **4** and repeat as many times as you want to.

6. Repeat **4** and **5** but this time, with the legs and arms wide apart.

7. When you are ready, catch hold of the insides of your feet with your hands. Bend your elbows and lower your head to the floor. Hold for a few breaths, slowly increasing the stretch.

8. Lift the head briefly and move the hands to the outsides of the feet. Repeat as in **7**.

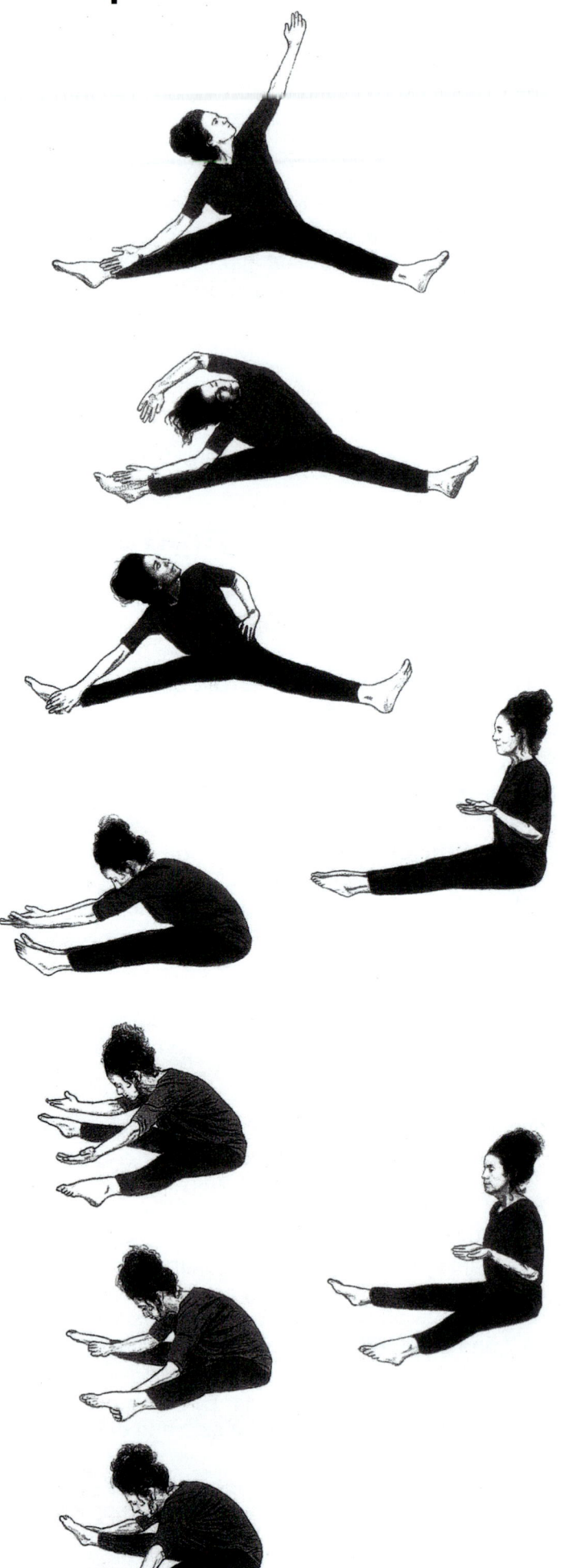

9. Sit with your right hip very close to the wall and the knees bent.
Twist round to the right and place your hands on the wall. Hold for a few breaths.

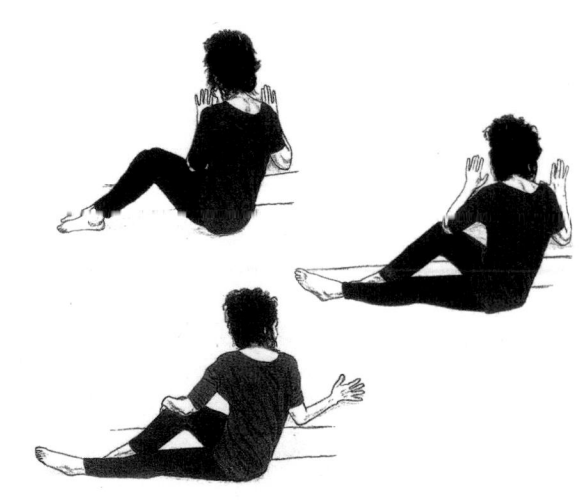

10. Straighten the left leg and twist round a bit more.

11. Place your left hand on your right leg and use it as a lever to increase the twist. Your right hand can slide out along the wall.
Hold for as long as you want to *and then change sides and repeat*.

12. Arrange your mat so that the top is touching the wall. Return to **9** and sit at the edge of the mat. With the hips very close to the wall, lower your back to the floor and use your arms and hands to swivel your back round and lift your legs up on to the wall. Your hips need to be as close to the wall as possible. Rest here for a few breaths.

13. Slide your feet down the wall, bringing the soles of the feet together and separating the knees, coming into **Cobbler on the Wall**. Sink as far down as you can so that the knees are wide apart.
Practise the **Pelvic Tilt** in this posture. First, tilt the tail bone down to the floor so that the lower back, under the waist, is slightly off the floor (as illustrated). Then tilt the tail bone upwards so that the lower spine pushes down into the floor. *Repeat a few times*.

14. Now increase the movement in the **Upward Tilt** by lifting the hips off the floor. Hold for a few breaths and then repeat the **Pelvic Tilt** a few times with the higher **Upward Tilt**.

15. Slide your right foot higher up the wall with the knee still bent but in line with the foot. Place your left foot over the right thigh.
Experiment, keeping the sole of the foot on the wall or pushing away with the toes.

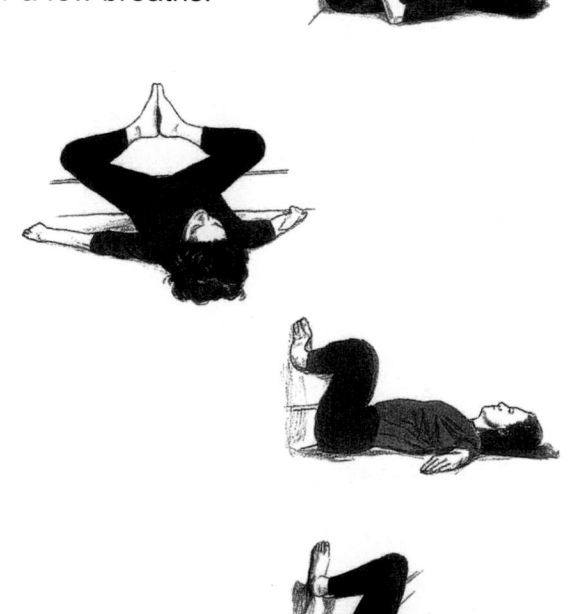

16. With the heel on the wall, lower the hips and move the left knee towards the wall. When you feel a stretch on the outside of your left hip you will know you have gone down far enough.

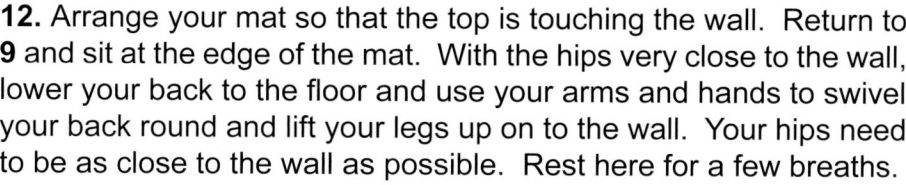

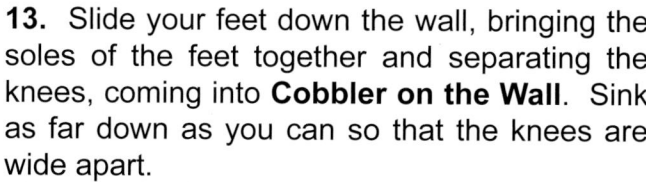

17. Hug your left knee into the chest.

18. Straighten the left leg over your head, holding it with both hands. You may choose to move the right foot a little higher. Hold for a few breaths, slowly increasing the stretch.

19. Take the heel off the wall and push away with the toes. Bend the elbows and pull the leg lower down.
When you are ready, return to 15, change sides and repeat.

20. Stand up and rest your hips and shoulders against the wall, with your legs at a 45-degree angle with the wall. It is important that you are standing on a non-slip mat. Bring your hands into **Prayer**.

21. Bend your knees and allow your back to slide down the wall. Carry on sliding until your thighs are parallel to the floor. You may need to adjust the position of your feet. Hold for a few breaths and then straighten the legs and slide back up the wall

22. Place your left foot over the right thigh and then slide down again. Proceed as in **21**.

23. Clasp your hands round your right knee and lift it as high as you can. Keep the hips forwards. Hold for a few breaths and then *repeat 22 and 23 on the other side*.

24. Bring your mat away from the wall and lie on it facing downwards. Slide your right knee up beside you as high as you can. Pass your left hand under the body and place it on the right knee. Swing your right arm back opening out the chest. The head can rest on the floor. Keep your right knee on the floor, look up and increase the twist to the left by moving the right shoulder away from the right knee.

25. Move into the **Flapping Fish**. A lot of people get confused when moving into this posture. If you are teaching it, either demonstrate it first or show pupils the illustration. Stretch your left arm above your head and rest your head on the upper arm. Bring your right shoulder and arm back, placing the right elbow on the right knee. Bend the left elbow and let the left hand rest on top of the right hand. Adjust your head so that it comes to rest on the hands or forearm. Make yourself comfortable and stay in this posture for as long as you want to. **Change sides and repeat 24 and 25.**

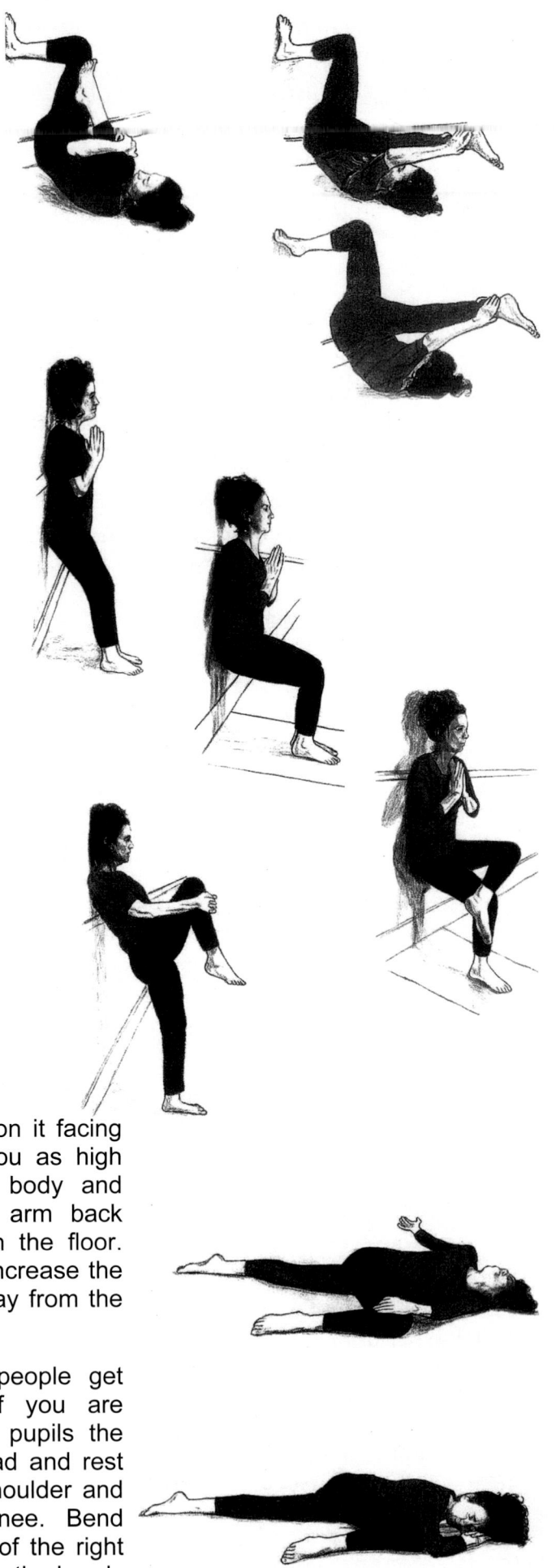

Faraday discovered Electromagnetic Energy (by means of induction[1]) in 1831 but, of course, it has existed since the beginning of time. It is a form of energy that can be reflected or emitted from objects travelling through space.

Some examples include gamma rays, x-rays, radiation, visible light, microwaves, radio waves and infrared radiation. None of these sound like good news for the human body but we could not exist without them. Most of our molecules interact weakly with electromagnetic fields in the radio frequency or extremely low frequency bands. One such interaction is absorption of energy from the fields which can cause tissue to heat up. More intense fields will produce greater heating.

Nerve impulses are electrical energy signals and they create energy fields and electromagnetic energy waves in the same way as when an electrical current is passed along a wire, it will create an electromagnetic energy field. Neurons create and control the electrical signals in the brain and nervous system. There are billions of these impulses in the body and these are constantly creating complex human magnetic fields. The human heart is a source of electromagnetism that can be detected by modern scientific instruments from a few metres away. The electrical energy waves the human body emits can be measured scientifically, infrared radiation being one that can be detected miles away with night vision equipment. If one tried to explain an aura, what better explanation than a subtle, luminous radiation surrounding a person.

Electromagnetic energy exists as attraction and repulsion of the poles. The neurones in our bodies have billions of electrical fields and poles attracting and repelling other poles. Might this explain romantic attraction and/or instant dislike?

Harnessing the power which obviously exists within us takes enormous strength of mind. Some selfless people summon their energies in an effort to heal others and often recipients say they feel heat (absorption of energy creates heat).

I am totally aware that I have learned to harness the power to help myself but only while researching this did I come to believe that the power I am using is electromagnetic energy. This has been achieved through belief and breathing practice.

If you ever doubt the power of magnetic energy, take a compass into a bomb shelter with 3ft thick walls. It will still point to the north. Gravity is responsible for the tides, our orbit round the sun and other orbits in our galaxy. This energy is still not fully harnessed by our poor, over-used planet. Electromagnetic energy is 10.64 times stronger than gravity and could be a source of natural renewable energy. It took from the origin of man until 1831 for Faraday to discover electromagnetic energy. Hopefully it will not be as many years again before we learn how to use it to its full potential.

Everything that ever was here is here now and always will be and all that we need for our future is all around us.

Written by Virginia Bonner-Davies, 2017.

Virginia (Gini) suggested I included this poem written by a friend of hers.

> This is a dot ——→ ·   What do you think of my dot? Not a lot I suppose, - but wait I beg and I will tell you of this dot, for it is a special dot. Its boundaries are the horizons of our knowledge and we exist within them.
> Little do we know that this dot be part of a sentence, or that the sentence be part of a book or the book be part of a library. All this and more do we miss wrapped up in our own little dot.
>
> By Peter Webb, c.1992.

1. **Induction** is a process where a conductor placed in a changing magnetic field (or a conductor moving through a stationary magnetic field) causes the production of a voltage across the conductor.

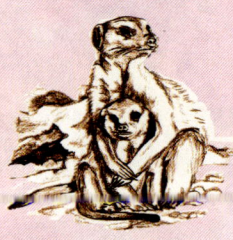
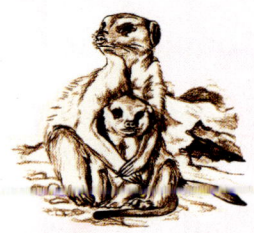

Heart Opening

This is divided into three sections: **1**. **Heart Stuff** and **Heart Fragments**. This is looking at the heart from a perspective influenced by recent scientific research. It will resonate with some people better than others. **2**. **Preparations** for the **Heart Opening Sequence**. **3**. **Heart Opening Sequence**.

Heart Stuff

The information and diagram in this section come from the **HeartMath Solution** by Doc Childre and Howard Martin (see **1** on the opposite page).

In the past few centuries, the idea that the brain in the head is the master organ in the body has taken hold. **In more distant times this distinction was given to the heart** and, thankfully, scientific research is leading us back to that perspective.

The heart is the first organ to form in the developing foetus. One of the great mysteries is the question of what triggers the first heartbeat. **It becomes like a caring parent** for the rest of the body as the organs develop in the womb. **After birth this continues**. The ancients understood this intuitively, now science is discovering the facts. It does much, much more than simply pump blood.

Messages are sent to the head brain via the Vagus nerve (associated with the Parasympathetic Nervous System, see page 12) and the Sympathetic Afferent Nerves. Information is sent to the Medulla at the base of the skull and then to the appropriate centres in the brain. Amongst other things, the heart sends signals that trigger the chemistry in the brain that is released into the body.

This is possible because the heart has its own independent nervous system. This is often called the brain in the heart. It has at least 40,000 neurons. Some are very similar to those in the head brain and **they can store memories**.

The heart is our gateway to the Universe. It has a very powerful electromagnetic field. At the time of writing, scientific instruments can pick up the extent of the heart's electromagnetic field **fifteen feet in every direction**. In the future, more sensitive instruments will find it extends further. Most things in the material world have electromagnetic qualities. This includes space, planets and stars. Human beings exist within and are a part of a Universal ocean of energy and information, which can be accessed by the human mind under the right circumstances.

To facilitate further understanding of the waves our heart creates, we need to define **Coherence**, **Incoherence** and **Heart Rate Variability**.

Coherence

In physics, two or more wave forms that phase-lock together so that their energy is constructive are described as coherent. It can also be attributed to a single wave form, in which case it denotes an ordered or constructive distribution of power content. When a system is coherent, virtually no energy is wasted because of the internal synchronisation among the parts. Think of a business or corporation that functions well and in which everybody thrives.

The heart is said to be in a coherent state when its components experience internal order and harmony. These are examples of emotions associated with this state: **happiness**, **appreciation**, **care** and **love**.

Incoherence

This is the opposite of coherence. This is like a business that isn't operating properly. There is disorganisation and lack of communication and harmony. These are examples of emotions associated with this state: **anger**, **frustration**, **unhappiness**, **hatred**, **despair and wanting to harm other creatures and things**.

Heart Rate Variability

HRV is the variation in the time interval between one heartbeat and the next. The heart rate changes from beat to beat, for example, when you **inhale** the heart rate **speeds up** and when you **exhale** it **slows down**.

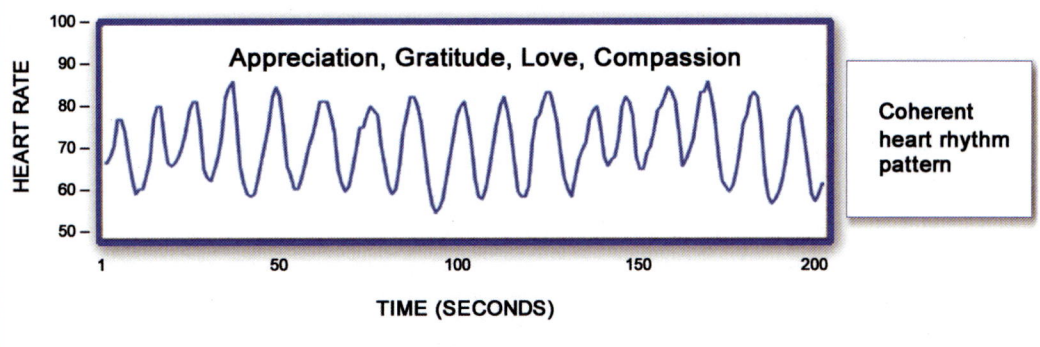

Positive Emotions and Heart Rate Variability

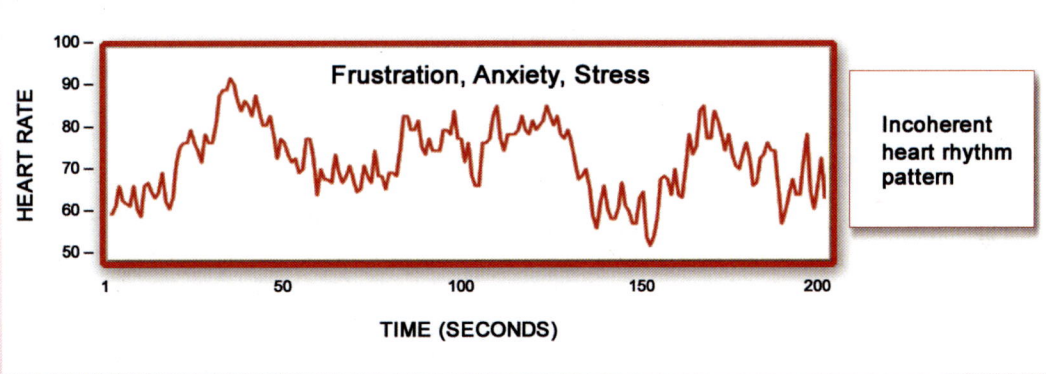

Negative Emotions and Heart rate Variability

Changing Heart Rhythms graphics used with permission from the HeartMath Institute
© 2017 HeartMath Institute

Heart Fragments

This refers to the next two pages.
Rather than write more pages of complicated information about the heart, I have placed fragments of information on appropriate backgrounds so that each fragment can be considered separately.

This information comes from three main sources:
1. **The HeartMath Solution** by Doc Childre and Howard Martin, published by HarperOne, 1999
2. **Waking the Global Heart** by Anodea Judith, published by Elite Books, 2006
3. **Videos** by Gregg Braden and the HeartMath Institute.

The background on the next page is of the sun rising over the River Ganges.
The opposite background is a painting of the Supreme Being in Paris in 1794 during the French Revolution. Robespierre set fire to a statue representing atheism and launched a new era of revolutionary virtue. The original painting is by Pierre Antoine Demachy. **Please note**, I will not attempt to hazard a guess at the quality of electromagnetic energy coming from this particular gathering of human hearts.
Both backgrounds come from *Man, Myth and Magic* magazines.

The heart's electrical field is about 100 times more powerful than the brain in the head and the magnetic field is 5,000 times more powerful [3]

Think of the heart as a radio transmitter broadcasting twenty-four hours a day. The quality of the broadcast is governed by every thought and feeling we have [1]

The human heart field interacts with and is affected by the electromagnetic field of the Earth, as well as other people, plants and animals [1]

Both intelligence and intuition are heightened when we learn to listen more deeply to our own hearts [1]

The heart sends more messages to the head brain than it receives from it [1]

If someone says to you,
"In the fortified city of the imperishable, our body, there is a lotus and in this lotus a tiny space: what does it contain that one should desire to know it?"

You must reply:
"As vast as this space without is the tiny space within your heart: heaven and earth are found in it, fire and air, sun and moon, lightning and the constellations, whatever belongs to you here below and all that doesn't, all this is gathered in that tiny space within your heart."
Chandogya Upanishad 8.1.2-3
8th to 6th century BCE

Opening your heart is like putting a wide-angle lens on the camera of your perception. Suddenly, more of the world comes into view. You have more room for new possibilities in the picture [1]

The emotional resonance you send from your coherent heart rhythms is like a magnet, attracting people, situations and opportunities [1]

The heart is in communication with our brain in every moment of every day. The higher the rate of coherence, the better the quality of the signal [3]

There are layers of the Earth's atmosphere, particularly the ionosphere, that happen to resonate within the same range of frequencies as our communications between our heart and brain. The ionosphere creates a symphony of frequencies [2]

The Institute of HeartMath was founded in California in 1991. Scientists and researchers from many different universities and walks of life, came together to explore the power of the human heart .

It is clear that our individual heart fields connect all of us together, the earth and space, in ways we don't yet fully understand.[1]

One of the main purposes of emotion in the human system is to provide a means of expression for core heart feelings.[1]

In the paradigm of the heart, the values of the divine feminine and divine masculine are held in relationship. It is not an either/or but a logical embrace of both, a balanced integration of I and thou... We need each other; we are enhanced by each other. Nature and civilisation, Earth and sky, matter and spirit, each are cosmic partners.... the sacred marriage of opposites.[3]

The rite of passage into the future is through an awakening of the global heart.[2]

Emotional energy works at a higher speed than thought. This is because the feeling world operates at a higher speed than the mind. Scientists have repeatedly confirmed that our emotional reactions show up in the brain activity before we have time to think.[1]

If we want to heal our bodies and create peace in our families and communities, we must speak to the fields that connect and find a meaningful language, a non-verbal language that communicates with the stuff the world is made of.[3]

Preparation for the Heart Opening Sequence

When you have mentally digested the revolutionary information about the heart, you can move on to the preparations for the sequence.

Without the mental orientation towards the heart, the **Heart Opening Sequence** would be no more than a chest-expanding or gentle backbend sequence. As such, most people will find the postures beneficial.

I find I can't have too many chest-expanding sequences. They are the necessary antidote to our slumped, seated, computer-orientated postures of the present times. They also mimic the body language of confidence and well-being, the opposite to the hunched postures of low self-esteem and depression. They are the feel good postures.

Lifting the head up and back will also be liberating and beneficial to most people but some caution is necessary. Some yoga teachers say, 'Never lift the head up and back'. This is limiting advice to the majority who do not find this movement problematic.

Caution

Please read Lisa Burato's comments on page 87 so that you are aware of the potential risks. Also, if you have neck problems, either leave out the backward bends or proceed with caution.

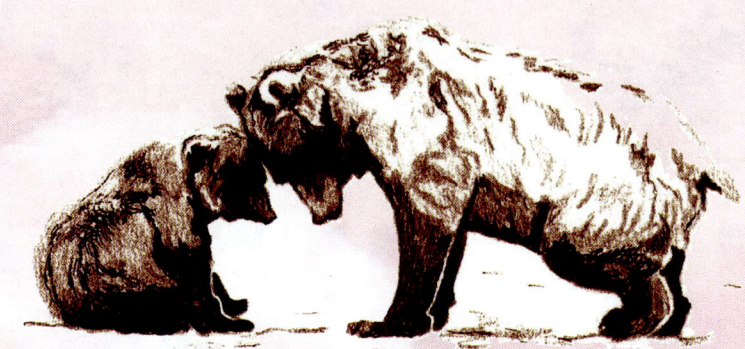

To facilitate the orientation towards and opening of the heart, I have included some suggestions made by David Frawley in **Yoga and the Sacred Fire**[1].

He unites the mantras **Om** and **Hreem** saying:

> ***Om** is the **Sound of the Infinite***
> ***Hreem** is the **Sound of the Heart***

> *Hreem is the mantra of the spiritual heart (Hridaya). It opens the small space within the heart in which the entire universe dwells. It is the source of the Divine Word, the unstruck sound that creates all things starting with space itself...*

> *Hreem is also the prime mantra of the Goddess or Divine Mother and brings us all her creative and transformative powers...*

> *The joint use of the two mantras OM and Hreem is the union of Shakti and Shiva, the cosmic masculine and feminine forces. You can use these two mantras together in order to unite the God and Goddess in your own heart as well as to contact their energy in the world around you...*

> *The unity of the sacred soul fire in the heart with the supreme light of consciousness is the essence of all knowledge.*

Method

Sit in any comfortable position and sing the mantras out loud a few times as suggested on the next page.

As you INHALE, intone (think) the mantra **Om** and direct your awareness and energy to the top of your head.

As you EXHALE, intone the mantra **Hreem**. Lower your awareness and energy through the **Throat Centre** into the spiritual heart.

Suggestions: I like to add, when the time is right, smiling emotional warmth down into the **Heart Centre** and visualising a flame (about the same size as a candle flame) flickering there.

Singing the mantras out loud

We are going to sing these two mantras out loud when we are practising some of the postures in the sequence. I was taught the following sentence when I took drama lessons at the Guildhall School of Drama while studying music there in the 60s.

Who would know aught of art must learn and then take his ease[2]

This is the Vowel Resonator Scale. It begins with the vowels that resonate at the back of your mouth, passes through the central vowels and then moves to the vowels that resonate at the front of the mouth.

Try singing **oo** as in **who**   and then   **ee** as in **ease**
Feel where the vowels resonate in your mouth/head

The mantra Om is usually sung starting with a short **ah** as in **art** (on a fairly low pitch). It is followed by **o** as in **of** (on a higher, but still in the middle to low range, pitch). Sometimes it is sung with an open **oh**, as in **home**.

At the beginning of the mantra the resonance goes to the back of the head. As you close the vibration with the consonant **m** as in **mouse**, the resonance comes down the front of your face to the nose and lips.

Hreem has a forward resonance as **ease** is the last word in the scale and **m** is the most forward nasal sound. This helps when taking the vibrations of the mantra **Hreem** to the **Heart Centre**. If you sing any vowel sound on a low pitch it will resonate in the chest but **eem** will resonate more naturally in the chest.
Try pushing the heels of your hands into the **Sternum** (the bone in the middle of the rib cage at the front). Take a deep **INHALATION** and sing **Hreem** on a medium to low pitched note. Press the hands into the sternum and feel the vibrations you are creating.

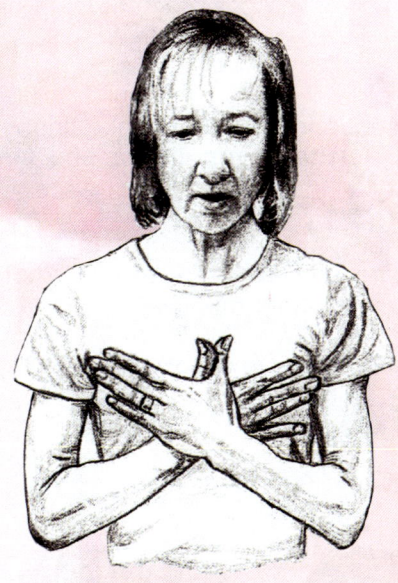

The position of the hands for feeling the vibrations in the **Heart Centre** when singing the mantra **Hreem**.

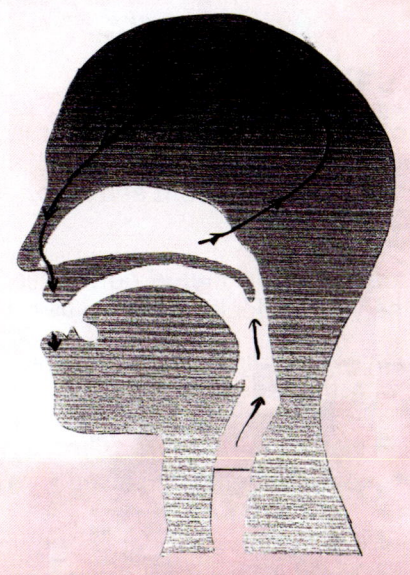

The path of resonance when singing the mantra **Om** or **Aum**. The lips will touch when you conclude with **mm**.

1. **Yoga and the Sacred Fire** by David Frawley (2004). Published by Lotus Press and Motilal Banarsidass Publishers PVT. LTD.
2. From **Voice Production and Speech** by Greta Colson (1963). Museum Press Limited. I am simplifying her interpretation of the **Vowel Resonator Scale** here to create an understandable concept of the resonance when singing the mantra **Om** or **Aum**.

Eye exercise

You will be doing this eye exercise in the **Upward Fish** posture in the sequence. You will need to practise it in a sitting position first.

Sit in a comfortable position, drop your shoulders and lift the chest, liberating the diaphragm. Stretch the top of the head to the ceiling, lengthening the back of the neck. Tuck in your chin a little and stick out your tongue. Try to keep the head as still as possible.

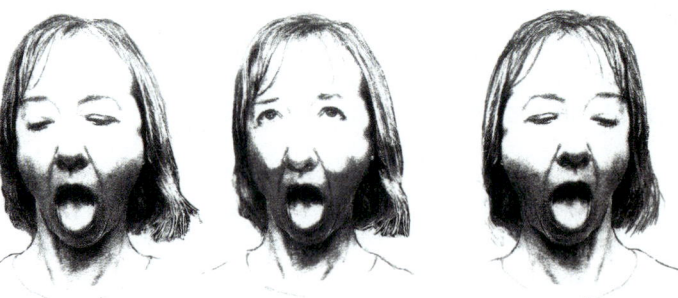

INHALE as you look up into the top of your head.

EXHALE as you look down to the left.

INHALE as you look up again.

EXHALE as you look down to the right.
Repeat as many times as you want to.

Observations

You can also practise this exercise with the head tilted slightly forwards and the neck in a more relaxed position.

In the context of the **Heart Opening Sequence** this exercise is symbolic. Before we can open our hearts we must open our minds. This may involve examining all our programmed belief systems and the fixed ideas that we carry around with us. We are often not aware of them or of the extent to which we are programmed, from childhood, to respond to the people around us and the environment we find ourselves in.

A quick glance through the history of humankind will teach us that we are very susceptible to brainwashing. We have believed some pretty extraordinary things. We may need to **open our eyes** and look at the world differently.

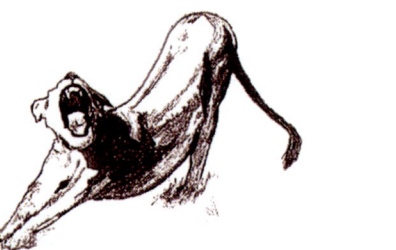

The Lion's Roar

You will also be making the **Lion's Roar** in the **Upward Fish**. In the sequence, we only make happy lion's roars but we will learn both happy and angry roars here as it will **further consolidate** and **simplify** your understanding of **Coherent** and **Incoherent Heart Rate Variability**.

1. Happy Roar

This is the roar of a lion that is not wasting energy. It is feeling secure and appreciative of Planet Earth. Imagine you are looking up at a beautiful full moon and the stars, in wonder and awe.

A. Sit on a chair or in **Easy Pose** on the floor or on a block, with the legs lightly crossed. Place your hands at the top of the thighs with the fingers spread out. Take a deep **INHALATION** through the nose with the mouth closed.

B. Open your mouth and stick out your tongue. Tilt your head slightly forwards, tucking in the chin and look up into the top of your head. **EXHALE** with a **happy Lion's Roar** and slide your hands down your thighs to the knees, stretching out your fingers as wide as you can.

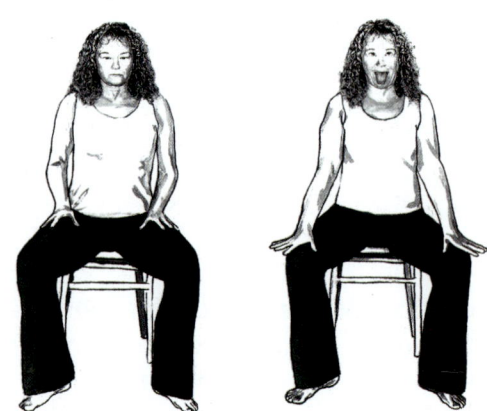

Observations

You will feel the roar in the chest and throat. It is the roar associated with the **Parasympathetic Nervous System** and **Ujjayi** breathing (see pages 10 & 37).
The message from your heart to the world will have a **Coherent Heart Rate Variability**.

2. Angry Roar

Imagine some hostile lions have been gradually encroaching on your territory. Now they are directly challenging you. You are feeling fierce, intimidated and angry. You are preparing to fight.

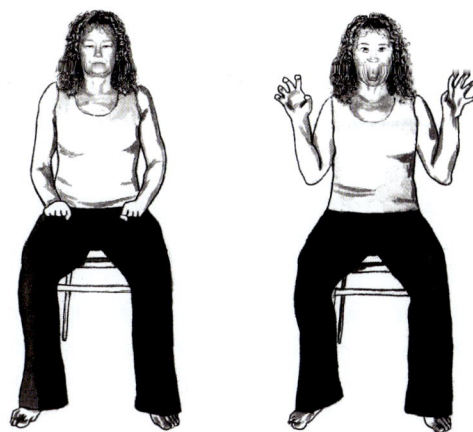

A. **INHALE** a lot of air quickly through your nose. Feel the nostrils being sucked together and the ribs lifting. Clench your hands on either side of the upper chest.

B. Open your mouth, stick out your tongue and **EXHALE** with an angry **Lion's Roar**. Move your hands up and out and use the fingers to mimic lion's claws. Lower the hands a short distance as you roar. Flare your nostrils angrily.

Observations

You will feel the roar at the top of the mouth and in your nose. It is associated with the **Sympathetic Nervous System**.

The message from your heart to the world will have an **Incoherent Heart Rate Variability**.

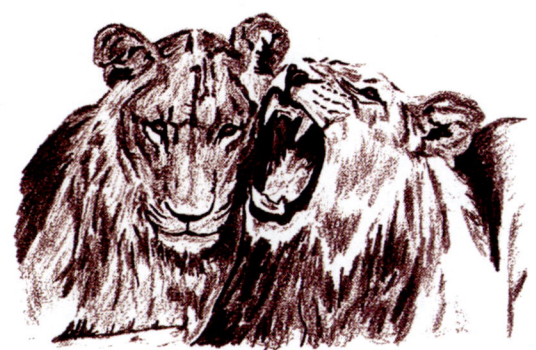

Additional notes

The idea for the **Lion's Roar** in the **Upward Fish** came from **Art of Sequencing**, **Volume Two**, **Seasonal Vinyasa** by Melina Meza (2011), Melina Meza Press. The inspiration for **1** and **11** in the **Heart Opening Sequence** also comes from this book.

Goddess Arms is also called **Cactus Arms** or **Goalpost Arms**. It is similar to the **Startle Response**. This is an arm movement you might make if you were suddenly startled by something, e.g., if you saw a rat or a snake you might raise your hands in horror. In this sequence the gesture has the opposite connotations. It is a gesture of celebration, harmony and empathy with all that is.

It is a sad fact that a lot of people don't enjoy singing these days. If you are practising the **Heart Opening Sequence** in a class you can vary the number of times you sing the mantras according to how much people enjoy singing them.

There are many scientific instruments on the surface of planet earth and orbiting it in space that track the electromagnetic frequencies coming from the planet. Spikes in activity were recorded on 11/09/2001 after the planes hit the World Trade Centre. There have been similar spikes during other global events, such as the death of Princess Diana.

The **Global Coherence Initiative** is an international effort that seeks to help activate the heart of humanity and promote peace, harmony and a shift in global consciousness. **GCI** conducts ground breaking research on the interconnectedness between humanity and earth's magnetic fields and energetic systems. For more information, search for **Global Coherence Initiative** on YouTube.

If you are feeling sceptical or confused by this information about the heart, there are many videos that may bring clarity. Try kicking off by searching for **Gregg Braden, Our Electromagnetic HEART Affects Reality** on YouTube. This will connect you to other relevant videos.

Other illuminating ideas can be found in **Spontaneous Evolution** by **Bruce H. Lipton PHD** and **Steve Bhaerman**, published by Hay House. ISBN 978-1-84850-305-2

Heart Opening Sequence

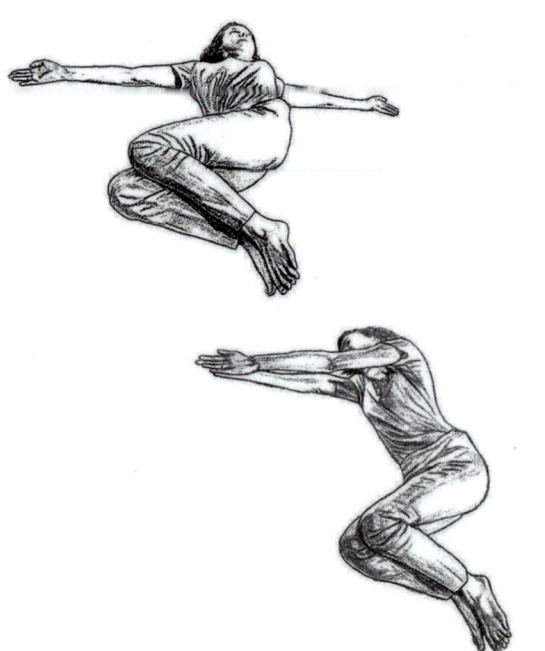

1. Lie on your back with your knees bent and the feet close together. Stretch your arms out to the side at a 180-degree angle, with the palms facing upwards. Move your hips a little to the left and lower your knees to the right. Push the left knee away from the left shoulder.
INHALE and feel the chest expanding and the heart opening.

2. EXHALE as you swing your left hand up and over your head. Turn to face the right and let the left hand rest in **Prayer** on top of the right hand. **INHALE** back to **1**.
Repeat a few times and then change sides and repeat.
You may choose to include **1** of the **Arm Circling Sequence** here.

Before attempting **3 - 5,** make sure you have practised the **Eye Exercises** and **Lion's Roars** in the preparatory section.

3. Stay on your back and straighten your legs with the feet together. Lift the upper body and place the forearms on the floor under your back, as illustrated. Point the toes and lift the chest. Let the head fall gently backwards (if this isn't comfortable, keep the head up) coming into the **Upward Fish**.

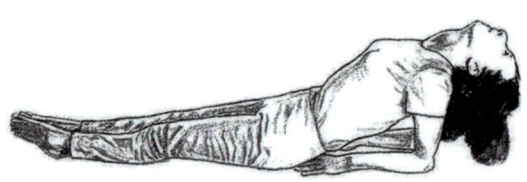

4. Open your mouth and stick out your tongue. Start the **Eye Exercise** as described on the previous page. Think about opening up the eyes of your heart. You will be **inhaling** as the eyes move towards the top of your head and the f oor and **exhaling** as you look up and out to the opposite sides.
Repeat as many times as you want to.
Sit up and lean forwards in between **4** and **5** if you feel you need to.

5. Make three **Happy Lion's Roars**. Feel appreciative and grateful. You can imagine you are roaring at a full moon and a beautiful night sky. Think about the message you are sending out to the universe from your heart. The electromagnetic waves will be coherent.

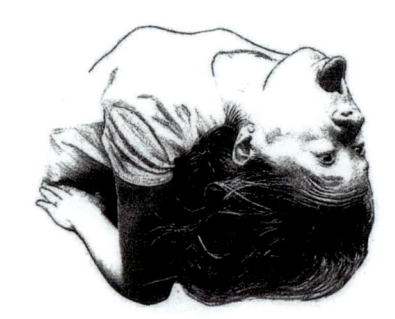

3. Slowly come to sitting. Place your hands behind you with the palms facing forwards. Bring the soles of the feet together and let your knees fall out to the sides. As you **INHALE**, expand the chest forwards and up. Allow the head to fall gently back.

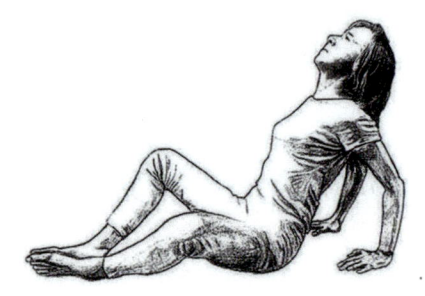

7. **EXHALE** as you bend your elbows more, tuck in your chin a little and stretch out your legs with the feet off the floor.

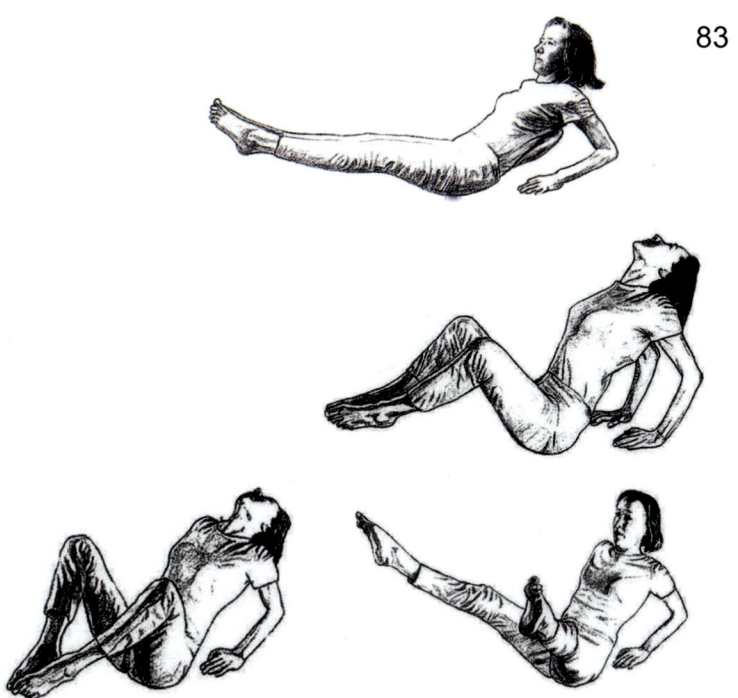

8. **INHALE** and return to **6**. This time, you can keep your feet off the floor.
Repeat as many times as you want to.

9. Return to **8** with the hands a little further apart. Repeat **7** and **8** a few times with the legs wider apart in **7**.

When you have practised **6 - 9** a few times you can start to add the mantras described in the preparatory section. A change in the breathing pattern will be needed to accommodate the extra **inhalation** needed before you sing **Hreem**.

Method
     INHALE into **6** or **8** and sing **Om**. The head need not be so far back.
     INHALE into **7** or **9** and then sing **Hreem**.

Observation: The chin will be tucked in a little as you sing **Hreem**. This will enhance the vibrations in the **Heart Centre**.

10. Move into **Animal Relaxation Pose** with your left lower leg on the outside of your left thigh and the right lower leg on the inside of the right thigh. The right foot is close to the body. Place your hands on the floor behind.
INHALE as you lift the chest and chin.
Pause for a few breaths as you bring your awareness to the elevated **Heart Centre**.

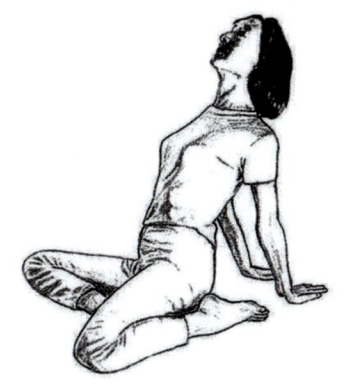

11. Bring your right foot out in front so that the right heel is in line with the left knee. Move your left heel in line with the left thigh. **INHALE** as you push up into a **Half Table Top Pose**. **EXHALE** as you lower the hips down, returning to **10**. Most people will find singing the mantras in **10** and **11** too demanding but some may choose to.
Repeat as many times as you want to before changing sides.

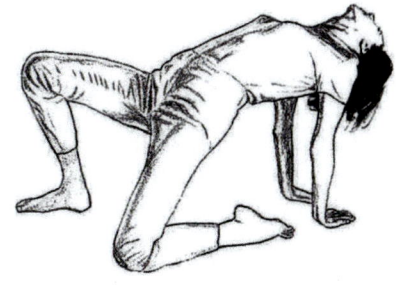

12. Come into a **Deep Lunge** with your right leg bent and the left knee on the floor and far enough back for you to feel a stretch along the top of the thighs. Bring your hands out in front with the palms facing but not touching.

INHALE as you swing them up over your head and look up at your hands.

EXHALE as you swing them out to the sides and back, down towards the floor and back to the starting position. This is only practised in one direction.

Continue to circle the arms round as many times as you want to.

Change sides and repeat.

For a variation you can go up on your back toes, coming into a **High Lunge**.

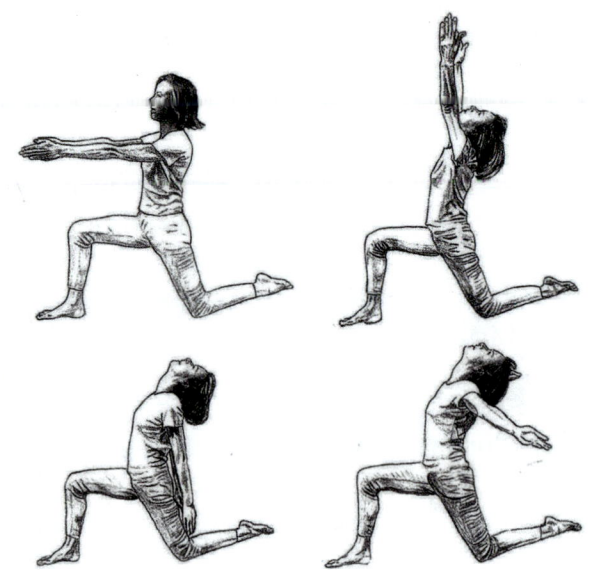

The Standing Section

No breathing instructions are given in this section. You can stay in the postures for as long as you want to.

13. Stand at the front end of your mat with the feet together. With the hands in **Prayer** position, sing a long resonant **OM**. Then place the heels of your hands on the sternum as described on page 70. Sing **Hreem** and feel the vibrations in the **Heart Centre**.

14. Catch hold of your elbows with your hands behind your back. Lift the chest and lean backwards. After a few breaths, come to an upright position.

15. Step backwards with your left foot.

16. Turn to the left to face forwards.

17. Lean backwards then return to **16**.

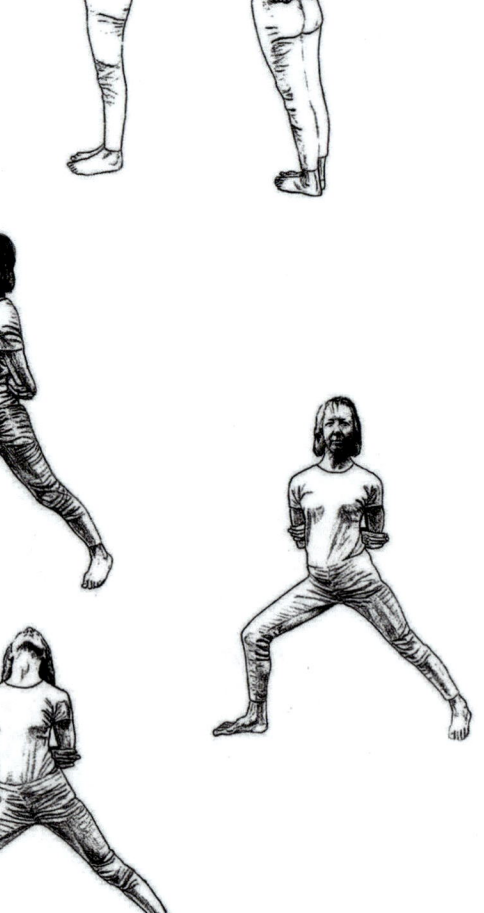

Please note, these postures mimic the **Warrior** poses but the thigh of the bent leg need not be parallel to the floor as is suggested in some schools of yoga. Here, the emphasis is on a different aspect of the posture.

18. Move into **Goddess Arms**. Please read the information about this in the **Additional Notes**. Bring the hands back forcefully, squeezing the shoulder blades together.

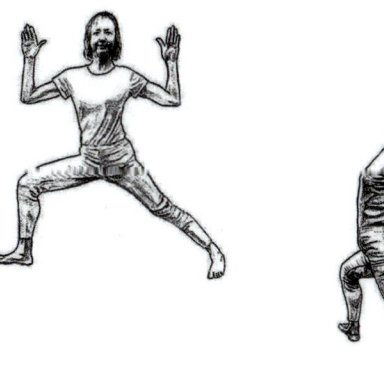

Sing OM

19.   Bring your hands behind your back and catch hold of your right wrist with your left hand.
Lean backwards and push your hands down to the floor, pulling your shoulders together. Feel the stretch on the front of your neck.

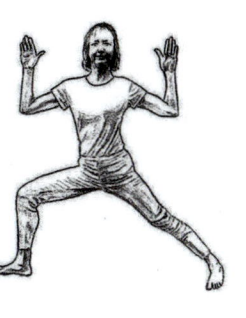

20. Return to **Goddess Arms**.

Sing Hreem

21. Bring your right elbow over your left elbow and wrap your arms around each other in **Eagle Arms**. This is also called **Garuda Arms**. If this doesn't suit your body type (if you have broad shoulders and short arms), cross your arms over on the chest with the hands on opposite shoulders. Lift the arms and lean backwards.

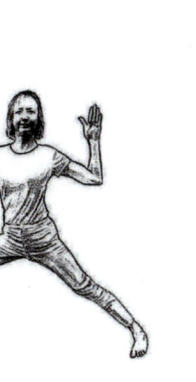

22. Return to **Goddess Arms**.

Sing OM

23.   Slide your right hand down the inside of the right leg and place left hand on the hip. Twist round, looking up to the left.

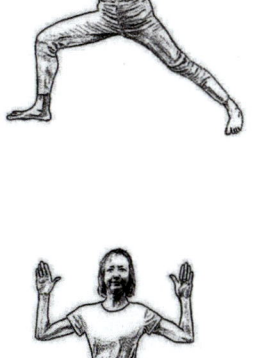

24.   Return to **Goddess Arms**.

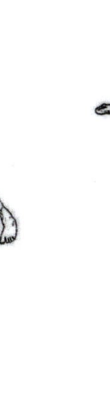

Sing Hreem

25.   Swing the hands back in **Flying Bird** and rotate over your right leg.

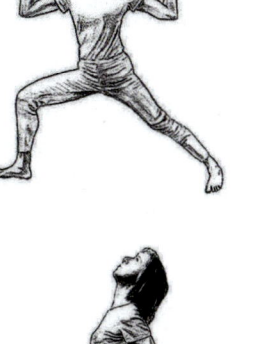

26.   Bring your left foot to the right foot returning to **13**. Sing the mantras again if you want to.
Repeat the Standing Section, changing to the right leg in **15**. Change the arms over in **19** and **21** and **23**.

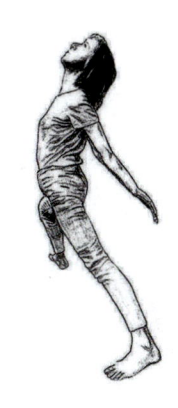
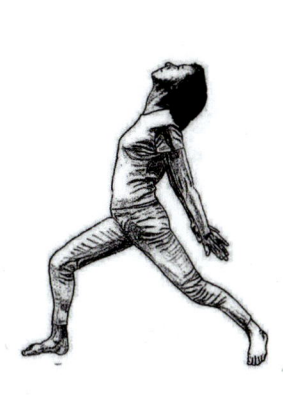
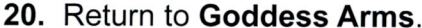

The Chair Section

Position the chair at the front or side of your mat with the seat facing towards you. It is best to have some of the chair on the mat so it can't slip.

27. The **Triangle** on a chair.
Face the chair and step forwards with your right foot so that it is as far under the chair as possible. The knee can touch the front of the chair. Step back with your left leg. The foot needs to be at a comfortable angle. Place your right forearm or hand on the chair and the left hand on your hip or stretch it up towards the ceiling.
Move the left shoulder back, rotating from the waist upwards and opening out the chest. Feel as if you are opening up your heart to the whole universe.
When you are ready, change the arms over and twist round to the right. You may go up on your back toes.
View your life from a different angle and open it to new possibilities and experiences.

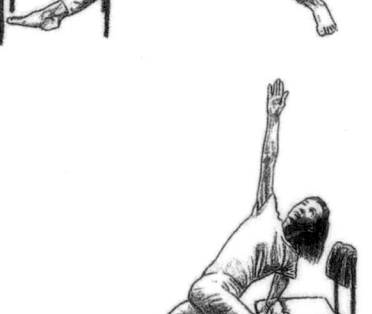

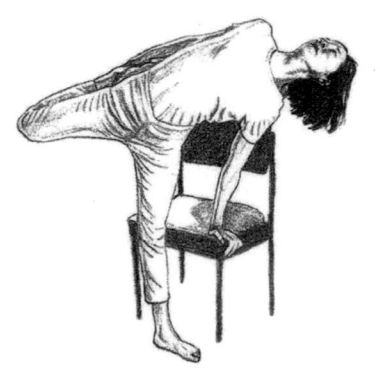

28. Stand with your left leg close to the chair and place your left hand on any very firm, secure part of the chair. Catch hold of your right foot with your right hand. You can start with the hand at the top of the thigh and slide it down the front of your leg to the top of your foot if you like.
Move your right shoulder back, bringing the hip and knee with it, and feel your wide, open heart.
Breathe compassion and empathy for all living creatures into the **Heart Centre** and radiate it to them when you breathe out.
Change sides and repeat.

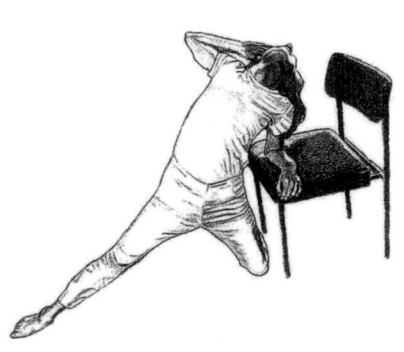

29. Kneel on your left knee with the lower leg in line with the chair seat. Place your left forearm on the chair and stretch out your right leg with the toes on the floor. Rest your right hand on the top of your head.
Move the right shoulder out to the side and back, opening out the whole of the right side of the body. Push away with the right toes.
As you experience this liberating stretch, think of John Lennon's song ***Imagine***. Think of all the best possible things that could happen to human beings and Planet Earth. Visualise a future where we live in peace and cooperate with each other. Imagine **coherent** heart energy saturating the planet.
After you have changed sides, visualise that the things you have just imagined have actually happened. Feel joyful and triumphant.

30. To conclude, sit on the chair with the hands in **Prayer**.
INHALE as you open out your arms wide and come into **Angel Wings**. Let your heart connect with the infinite energy of **Creation** and its **Source**.
Bring your wings together in front and send love and compassion to all sentient beings on Planet Earth (humans, animals and anything that experiences feelings).
Bring your hands into **Prayer** and sing a final **OM** and **Hreem**.

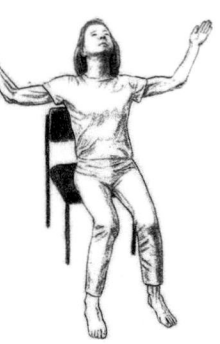

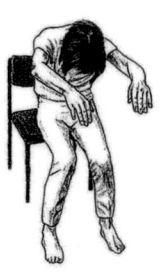

The Necessity for Caution when Putting the Head Back

The neck is composed of seven vertebrae stacked upon each other to provide support and movement to the head. This arrangement provides flexibility and a lot of movement to permit correct positioning to the sense organs in space (eyes, ears, nose and mouth). The neck also carries major vital structures to and from the brain to the body. Important arteries and veins, air pipes and nerves commanding movements of the body and its vital functions, are carried in the neck with hardly any major structural protection surrounding them. This is because a hard and bony cage would mean loss of range of movement that is so necessary in this anatomical region.

It is important therefore to understand the relationship between maintaining a healthy level of movement and flexibility of function of the neck, whilst being very careful and mindful of these vital structures passing between joints and underneath muscles.

Accidents, falls and genetic abnormalities cause the neck to become even more vulnerable to instability and possible compression of nerves and vessels. When exercising it is therefore paramount to listen to one's body. Signs like dizziness, light-headedness, visual changes, tingling or numbness in the limbs, sharp pain or difficulty swallowing are major red flags and indicate that you need to swiftly stop any exercise and seek medical help.

If you have suffered with previous neck issues, car accidents, vertigo when turning the head, or are taking medications, it is advisable to ask your GP for advice before starting any exercises, especially when they involve arching and/or deeply rotating the head backwards. This particular combination of movements – backward arching and rotation of the neck – put strain and compression on one of the vessels taking blood to the brain, the vertebral artery. This artery is very easily injured with very unpleasant consequences, including strokes.

It is therefore very important to keep in mind this gentle structure when exercising and doing this particular set of movements and, if in doubt in regard to the health of your neck, avoid them altogether until you have consulted a health professional.

A great way to get the benefits of this practice without physically engaging in the techniques is to mentally visualise and perform each movement in your mind's eye. Imagine and **see** your body going through the full sequence. Spend the same amount of time **observing** your body freely doing each of the listed movements and **hold** the pose for the suggested times. This will give you very similar benefits without any of the possible complications.

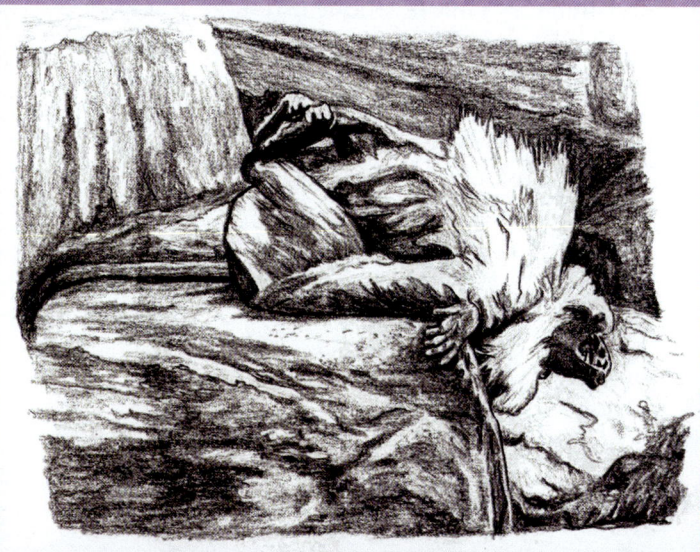

However, it is important not to become too fearful to use the body in healthy and expressive ways. Therefore, before limiting your practice with unnecessary worries, do consult a GP and ask their permission to perform the postures in the **Heart Opening Sequence** and just be gentle and mindful with your movements.
Good luck with your practice!

Elisa Burato M.Ost.
kuulondon.co.uk

A baboon hanging with its head back over a ledge.

Aphantasia

Although I use visualisation frequently in my classes, I have only recently discovered that some people can't visualise. I was driving home down twisty country lanes listening to Radio 2[1]. I had just been doing a **So Hum** class with my 95 year old pupil. We had been counting sheep coming through a hole in a fence at the end of the class. On the radio a man called Neil spoke about a childhood experience when he discovered he couldn't visualise counting sheep.

'My stepfather, when I couldn't sleep, told me to count sheep, and he explained what it meant. I tried to do it and I couldn't. I couldn't see any sheep jumping over fences. There was nothing to count.'

Neil admits some aspects of his memory are 'terrible', but he is very good at remembering facts. He struggles to recognise faces but he does not see aphantasia as a disability, simply a different way of experiencing life.

Research on the Internet revealed people like Tom who didn't realize he had the condition until he was 21. He says it makes him feel isolated. Tom says, *'The ability to recall memories and experiences, the smell of flowers or the sound of a loved one's voice: before I discovered that recalling these things was humanly possible, I wasn't even aware of what I was missing out on.'*

Aphantasia is the suggested name for a condition where one does not possess a functioning mind's eye and cannot visualise imagery. The phenomenon was first described by Francis Galton in 1880[2]. It remained largely unstudied until 2005. Professor Adam Zeman of the University of Exeter was approached by a man who seemed to have lost the ability to visualise after undergoing minor surgery. The team led by Zeman published its findings in 2015. They coined the term *aphantasia*.

It is similar to invisible disabilities such as colour blindness, face blindness, word blindness, and tone deafness. A definition of aphantasia is where a person is unable to synthesise senses in their mind. It appears to be a spectrum condition where the degree of Aphantasia varies. Certain people are unable to create any images, sounds, tastes, smells or touch within their mind. This is known as **Total Aphantasia**.

Professor Zeman is adamant that aphantasia is 'not a disorder' and says it may affect up to one in 50 people. If you think you have aphantasia or its exact opposite, **hyperphantasia**[3], and would like to be involved in Professor Zeman's research, he is happy to be contacted at: a.zemen@exeter.ac.uk

If you would like to complete a questionnaire to find out if you have aphantasia, go to: http://aphant.asia/have-i-got-aphantasia

I taught at Inglewood Health Hydro for five years before it was taken over for a housing development. Myself and other teachers found that strange healing experiences happened there. It used to be a monastery. After a yoga class which I had ended with Betty Shine's Self Healing meditation/visualisation, a lady in her 30s or 40s came up to me and said that that was the first time in her life that she had ever been able to visualise. I didn't think any more about it until learning about aphantasia.

In another twist in the visual jigsaw puzzle, my son came across a YouTube video in which a lady who had been blind from birth had a near-death, out of body experience. She could see the doctors and what was going on around her with normal vision. The link is: Near Death Experience-Blind woman sees while out of body-You Tube

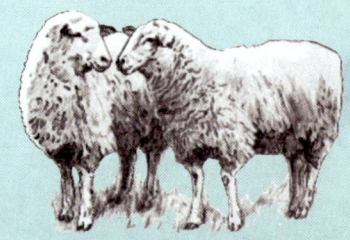
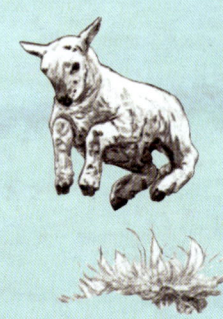

1. www.bbc.co.uk/news/health-34039054
2. *'To my astonishment, I found that the great majority of the men of science to whom I first applied, protested that mental imagery was unknown to them, and they looked on me as fanciful and fantastic in supposing that the words 'mental imagery' really expressed what I believed everybody supposed them to mean. They had no more notion of its true nature than a colour-blind man who has not discerned his defect of the nature of colour.'*
3. The super-visualiser. Read about the children's book illustrator Lauren Beard on the BBC website quoted in 1.

Sung Meditations

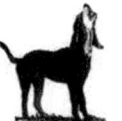

I was taught this Kirtan Kria by Darryl O'Keeffe at a workshop. Yogi Bhajan, who formed the Kundalini Yoga Movement, developed this meditation. I have simplified it to use at the end of my yoga classes. To access the original version type 'Kirtan Kria, Sa Ta Na Ma' into your search engine.

Sa - the universe, totality
Ta - life, creation
Na - death, dissolution
Ma - rebirth, regeneration

Sing the mantra slowly using this melody at your chosen pitch.

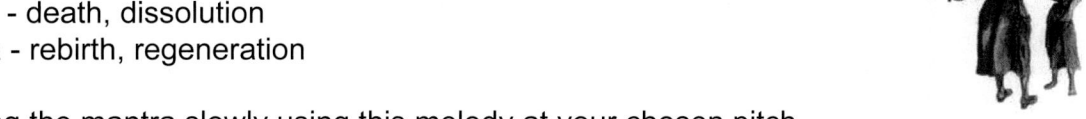

There are four sections. You can pace these according to the time available and your inclination.

1. Sing it about twelve times. Roughly four times very loudly, four times at middle volume and then again softly, gradually reducing the volume until you can hardly hear it.

2. Repeat (intone) the mantra silently for as long as you choose to.

3. Start to sing the mantra again about the same number of times as in 1, but reverse the volumes. Start very softly, move to middle volume and finish very loudly.

4. Repeat the mantra silently again.

Two other mantras suit this format well:
Om Mani Padme Hum. This is a Buddhist chant, often translated *Hail the jewel of the lotus flower*.

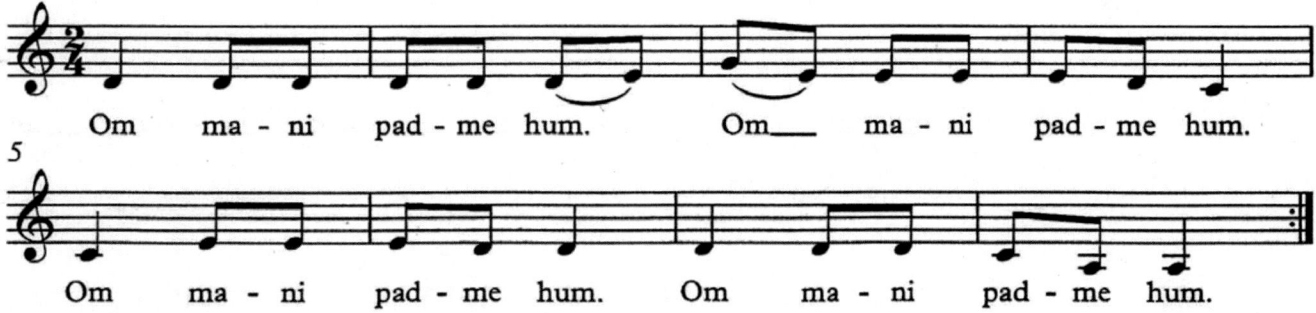

Shri Ram, Jai Ram, Jai Jai, Ram Om. Ram is short for Rama. Lord Rama is considered by Hindus to be an incarnation of God. His heroic life story is told in **The Ramayana**.
It translates, *Lord Ram, Hail* or *Victory to Ram*. **Om** is known as the universal sound.

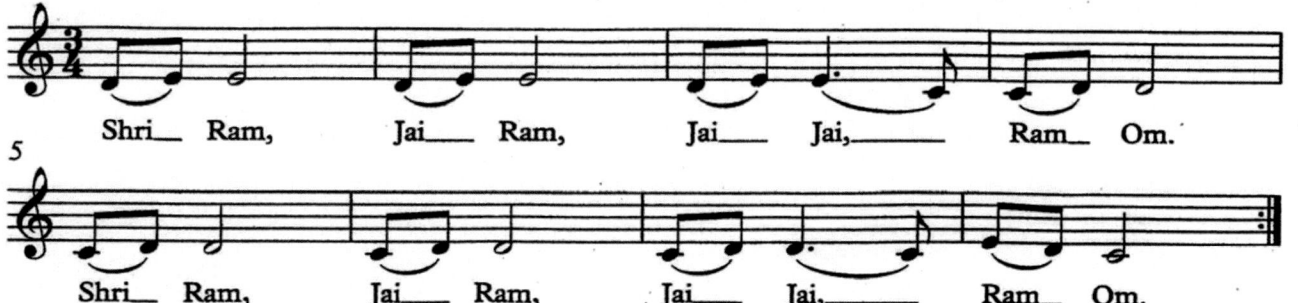

So Hum Class

Meditating in the Postures

I did my first **So Hum Class** while staying at the beautiful Mandala Ashram in south Wales many years ago. It made a great impression on me and I have taught variations of it to my pupils on a regular basis. It will be my weekly class about every four months. It has evolved over the years. I have experimented with other two-syllabled mantras but always return to **So Hum**. This is usually translated to mean, *I am that I am.*

I start with standing postures and include a few simple balancing ones. These are mostly adapted from the very resourceful book, *Tree Yoga*[1]. As the class progresses and we become more relaxed, we descend to the floor. I always include the **Canoe Sequence** from my previous books. I have repeated it here with suggestions for adapting it for this class. I vary the rest of the class. Uncomplicated sequences and postures with lots of repetition work well.

We aim to establish the state of **Pratyahara,** the withdrawal of the senses (see **Glossary**). We say, 'Bye, bye planet Earth' for the duration of the class. Try to keep your eyes closed as much as possible. During some of the balancing postures you will need to open your eyes.

As you become more and more relaxed, you may automatically find yourself using **Ujayi breathing**, see page 39. When I hear lots of *throat breathing,* I know my pupils are deeply relaxed and the class is working its magic. Most of the time, make your **exhalations** longer than your **inhalations**.

The Method

We are going to intone[2] the mantra for the entire class, even when we are resting or pausing between postures.

> Think **SO** on every **INHALATION**
> and **HUM** on every **EXHALATION**

1. Start by sitting and singing the mantra a few times. Here is a suggestion for a melody. Swami Saradanada sang a similar melody in a workshop.

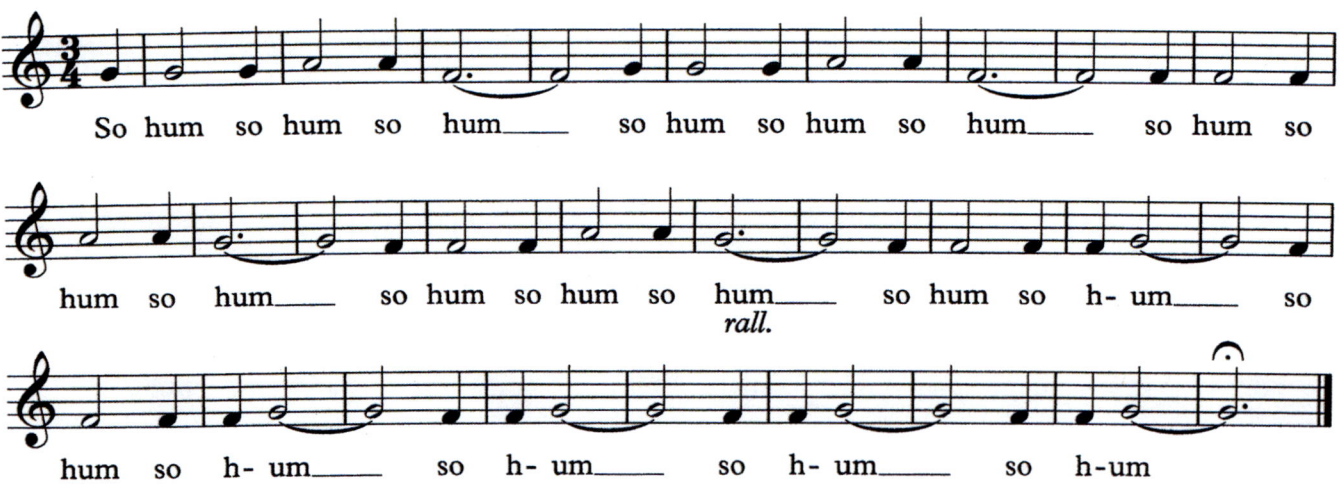

2. Lie on your back with your hands behind your head and the hands and feet wide apart. Point your toes.

INHALE (think **SO**) and as you **EXHALE** (think **HUM**), stretch your fingers away from your toes. **x2.** The third time, hold the stretch for a few breaths (as always, repeating your mantra).

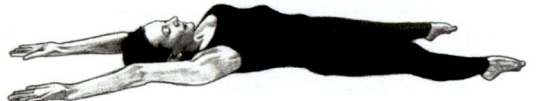

1. **Tree Yoga** is by the Kundalini Yoga teachers Satya Singh and Fred Hageneder. Published by Earthdancer GmbH, 2007.
2. Intone is a term used to suggest thinking or internalising a mantra. Sometimes I say 'think' as some people may relate to that more easily. The important thing is to appreciate the special vibration of your mantra.

INHALE as you tense
EXHALE as you release

INHALATIONS
SO

EXHALATIONS
HUM

Tense your toes and your feet.
Release.

Bring your toes back towards your head.
Release.

Tense the buttocks.
Release.

Sink the hollow of your back into the floor
and flatten the abdomen.
Release.

Tense the upper back and the chest.
Release.

Clench your fists tightly, lift your hands a little
off the floor and bring your shoulders to your
ears. *Hold and breathe with your mantra
for at least 4 breaths. Release.*

Lower your hands. Stretch your fingers out
wide and push your shoulders and fingers
down towards your feet.
Hold as above. Release.

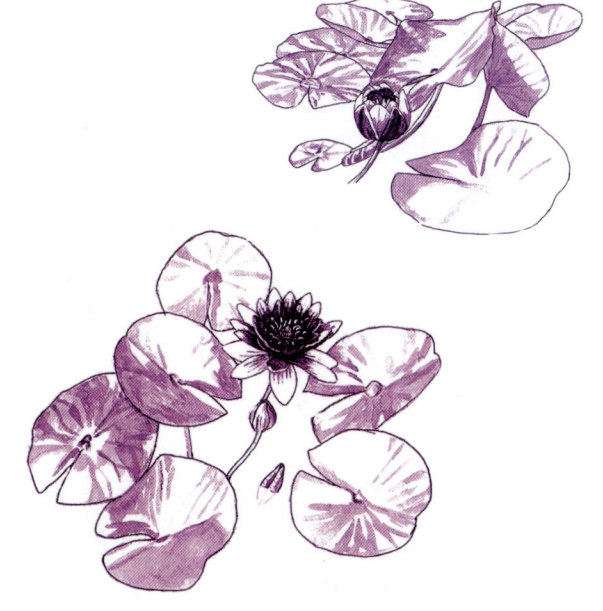

Roll your head to the right as you **INHALE** and think **SO** and **EXHALE** it slowly to the left as you
think **HUM**.
Repeat a few times.

4. To further connect to the mantra, place your hands on the abdomen. Breathe with a completely
relaxed abdomen. Think the mantra loudly a few times to reinforce it. Eventually it will establish
itself in your mind. It will drift through your awareness like waves in the sea. Sometimes it will be a
little wave and sometimes a more energetic one.

Feel the abdomen rising under the influence of the diaphragm when you **INHALE** and flattening
as the diaphragm moves up into the rib-cage when you **EXHALE**.

After about 8 breaths, start to pause after the **inhalation** and **exhalation**. This empty,
hollow, timeless space is very special. It is to be treasured and cultivated. Sow timeless seeds of
emptiness there. When you stop breathing, you stop thinking. You can pause for about 8
seconds, but don't count because then you are using words.

5. When you feel the time is right, roll over onto your right hand side and come to sitting. Sit in
Easy Pose, your chosen meditation posture or on a chair.

INHALE as you imagine a bright, silvery white
healing light entering your head between
your eyebrows.

EXHALE as you visualise this loving,
peaceful light and energy leaving the top of
your head.

When you concentrate on the front of your head
you may pick up a high-pitched electronic
sound. For more information, go to page 115.

The Standing Section

6. When you feel the time is right, stand up slowly.
Stand with the feet a hip-width apart. Lower your head until the trunk is parallel with the floor. Stretch your hands out behind you with the palms facing upwards. The chin may be forwards or in a neutral position.

INHALE as you stretch your fingers out wide.

EXHALE as you clench your fists. *Repeat at least 5 times*.

Close your eyes if possible and turn your senses inwards, as always in this class.

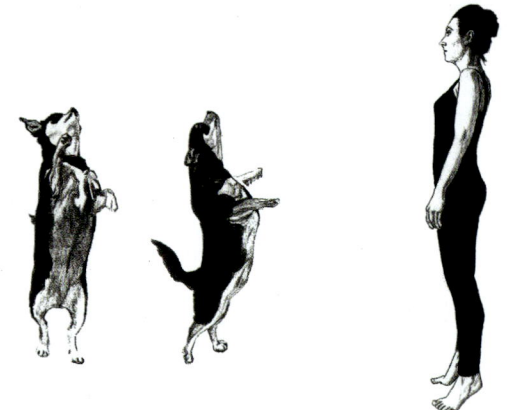

8. The **Standing Cat**
Stand with the feet a hip-width apart and place your hands on your bent knees.

INHALE into **Upward Cat**.

EXHALE into **Downward Cat**.

Repeat as above.
You may choose to reverse the breathing pattern.

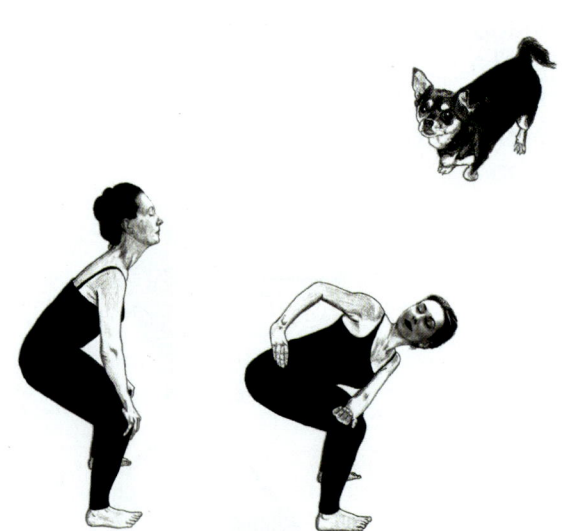

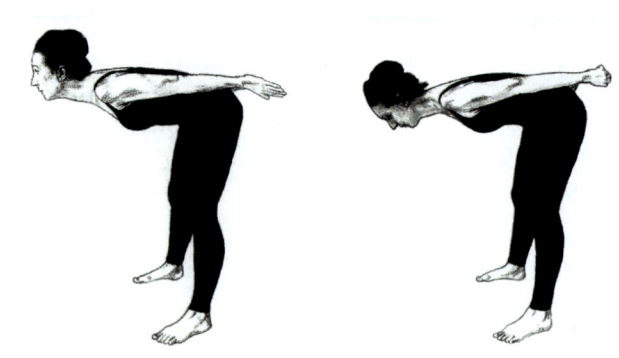

7. Stand with your feet together or a comfortable distance apart. Let your hands hang loosely by your sides. Tuck in the tail bone and stretch the top of your head towards the ceiling.

INHALE as you rise up on tiptoes.

EXHALE as you lower your heels to the floor.

Continue for your chosen number of breaths.

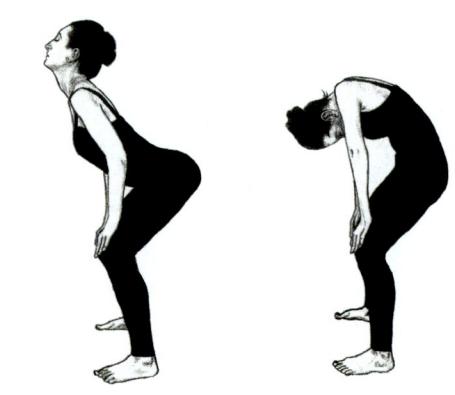

9. Begin in the same posture as in **8** but the spine can be in a more neutral curve.

INHALE with the elbows straight.

EXHALE as you lower your left elbow to the left knee. Place your left hand on the right knee with the palm facing upwards. With your right hand on your hip, twist round to the right.

INHALE back to the centre and **EXHALE** to the left.

Change sides and repeat.
You can vary it by pausing for a few breaths in the twists, repeating the mantra as always.

10. With the feet still a hip-width apart, place your fingers on your shoulders.

INHALE as you lean backwards. Open out the chest and bring the shoulder blades together. Let the head fall back if it is comfortable.

EXHALE as you bring the elbows and forearms together in front. Tuck in the chin and tailbone as you round your back.

Repeat as desired.

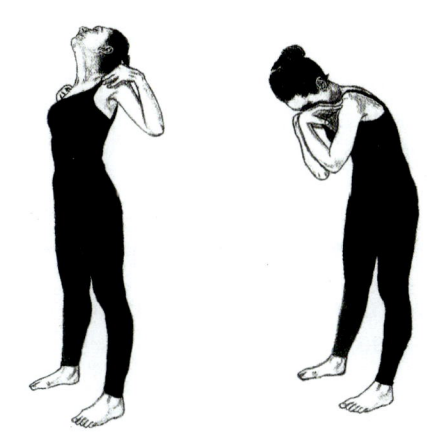

11. With the palms facing, clench your fists.

INHALE your arms up in front, bending at the elbows. They need not touch.

EXHALE as you swing your elbows out to the sides. The fists face downwards.

Repeat as above.

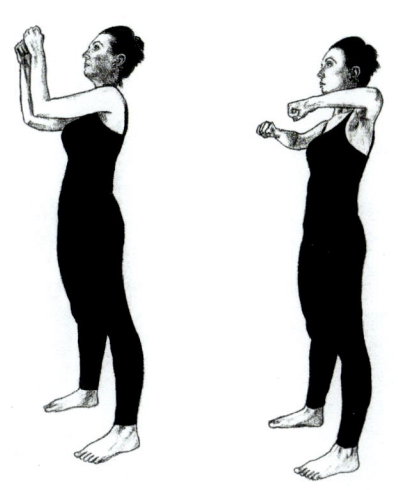

The Balancing Section

12. Place your right hand under the left armpit. Let your left hand hang loosely.

INHALE as you swing your left leg forwards.

EXHALE as you swing it back. The foot should not touch the floor.

Repeat about 8 times and then change sides and repeat.

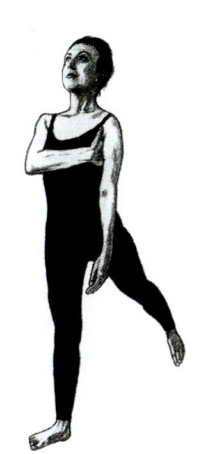

TIPS FOR BALANCING
Spread the toes out on the foot that you are balancing on and imagine that your big toe is Super Glued to the floor. Sometimes I just say Super Glue and my pupils know what I mean,

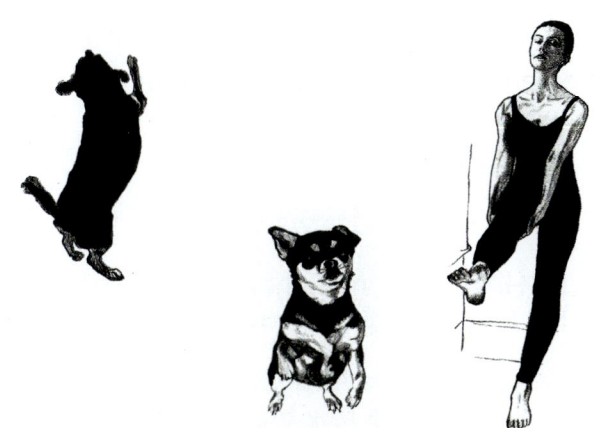

13. Stand with your hips against a wall and your feet a comfortable distance from the wall. Lift your right leg and point your toes. Place your hands on or under your leg. Close your eyes, as usual, and connect deeply to your mantra.

When you feel the time is right, change sides and repeat.

14. Move back to your mat and lift your left leg behind you. Point your toes and place your hands on the right knee.
Hold and repeat as in 13.

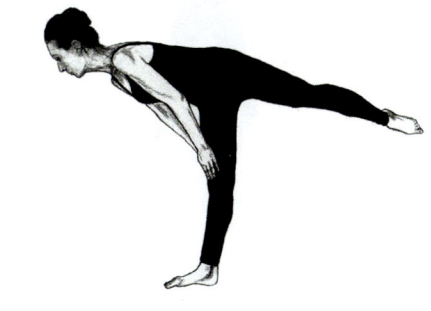

15. Start with your feet together.

Lift your left leg out to the side and bring the toes towards the head.

Stretch your right arm out to the side with the palm facing downwards.

Place your left hand on the right thigh.

Hold for a comfortable duration and then change sides and repeat.

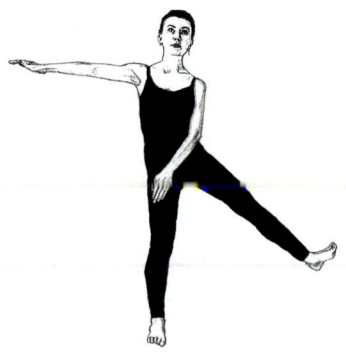

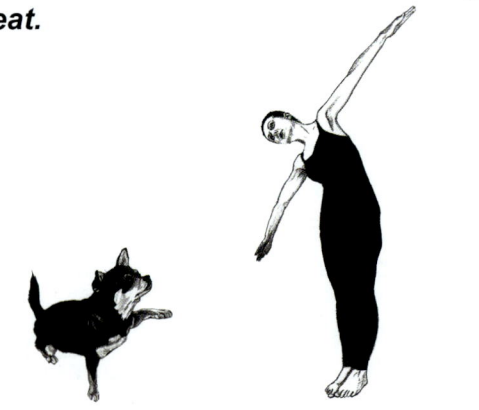

16. Stand with the feet together.

Stretch your hands out to the sides with the palms facing downwards.

Maintain a 180 degree angle and push the fingers away from each other.

Lower down to one side, as illustrated.

Hold and repeat as in **15**.

17. Move the feet wider apart. With the arms raised and bent, bring your thumbs and first fingers together.

INHALE as you face forwards.

EXHALE as you twist round to the right. You can change the angle of your back foot or go up on your toes if it is more comfortable.

Continue as in **9**, either *change sides and repeat* or *pause and breathe in the twists*.

18. You can repeat **17** with your hands out to the sides.

19. Interlock the hands in **Ksepana Mudra** (see page 49). Make a large circle with your hands. When your hands are forwards, your hips will be backwards and vice versa.

> **To coordinate the breath** with the circling movements, **INHALE** as the body opens up, i.e., when the hands move up and back, and **EXHALE** as the body closes up, when the hands lower. As usual, try to make the exhalations longer than the inhalations.

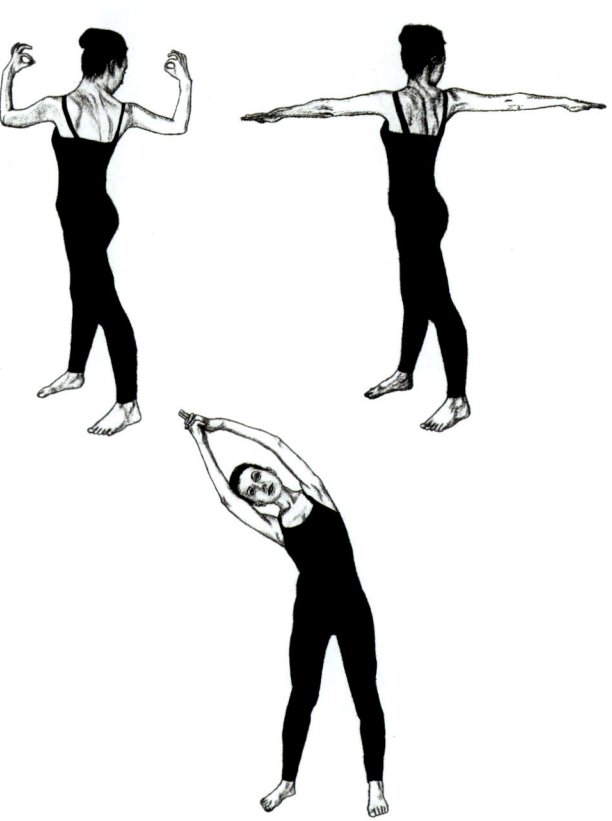

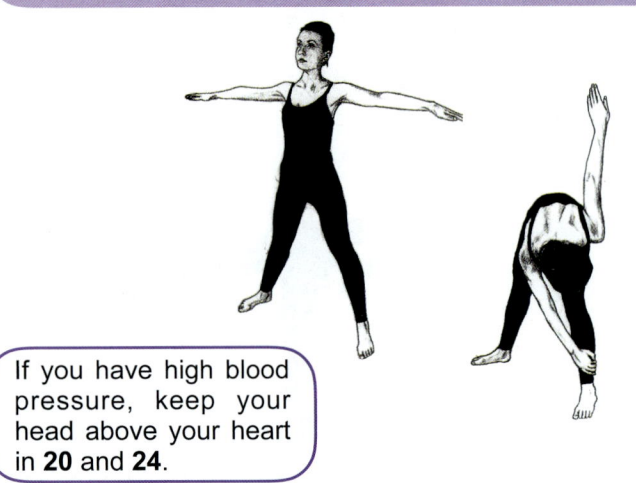

> If you have high blood pressure, keep your head above your heart in **20** and **24**.

20. Move lengthways on your mat with the feet wider apart.

INHALE the hands out to the sides with the palms facing downwards.

EXHALE the right hand down to the lower left leg. Lift your left arm up to the ceiling.

Either *change sides and repeat* or *hold the twist for a few breaths*, as in **9** and **17**.

You can increase the twist by holding the leg firmly with the opposite hand, bending your elbow and lowering the shoulders.

21. Bend your knees and sink into a **Half Squat**. The hands can be in front, as illustrated, or higher with the thumbs and index fingers touching.
Hold and breathe with your mantra.

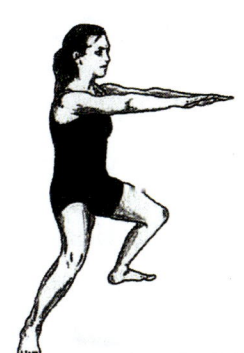

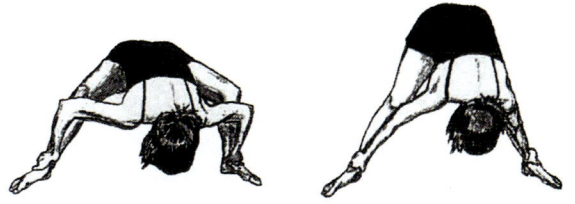

If you have high blood Pressure, compromise by placing your hands on the seat of a chair in **22** and **23**.

22. Place your hands on your ankles. **INHALE** as you bend your elbows and sink into a deep squat. **EXHALE** as you straighten your legs and arms. *Repeat as many times as you want to.*

23. Bringing your feet together, go up on your toes. Place your fingertips on the floor in front, as illustrated. **INHALE** in the squat and **EXHALE** as you straighten your legs and arms. *Repeat as in 22.*
You can hold the upward posture, pushing up on your fingertips and toes, for a few breaths to conclude.
This is the **Frog** as taught in **Kundalini Yoga**.

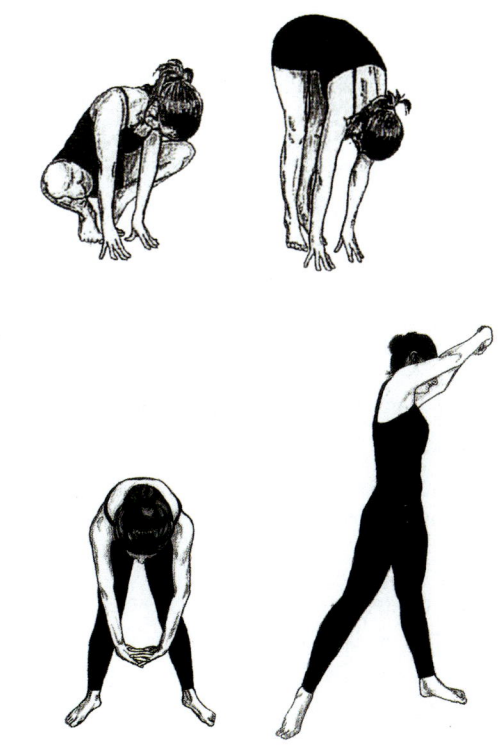

24. With the feet wider apart, bring your hands into **Venus Lock** or **Ksepana Mudra**.

INHALE with you hands held in front, at waist level or lower.

EXHALE as you go up on your right toes and swing your hands up to the left.
Push up on your toes and twist round as far as you can.

Continue as in 20.

25. Finally, **The Stationary Walk**. This is inspired by **Dru Yoga**. One foot stays in the same place while the other foot steps backwards and forwards. The arms follow the moving leg.

Start with the feet together and the hands by your sides.

INHALE as you step forwards with your left foot and swing your arms up. You can go up on the right toes.

EXHALE as you step backwards with the left foot and swing your arms back. You can go up on your right heel.

Continue for about eight breaths then change sides and repeat.

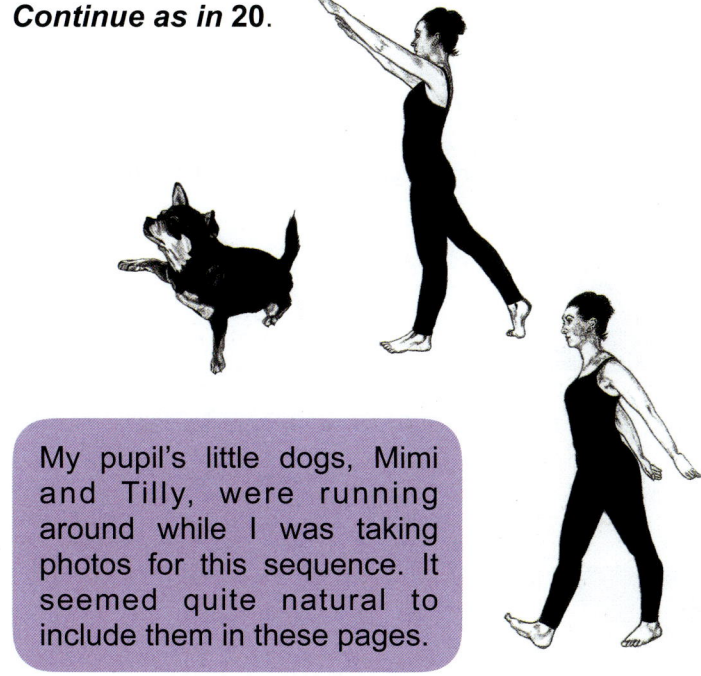

My pupil's little dogs, Mimi and Tilly, were running around while I was taking photos for this sequence. It seemed quite natural to include them in these pages.

The Canoe Sequence adapted for a So Hum Class

This sequence adapts well for a So hum class. The procedure continues:

Keep your eyes closed whenever possible
Intone So on the **inhalation**
and **Hum** on the **exhalation**

1. Lie on the floor, face downwards, with the hands stretched out in front. Every time you **EXHALE** push the fingers away from the toes. For about **5** breaths.

> The chin can be up or down in all the postures except for those where the head is resting on a hand (7 – 10).

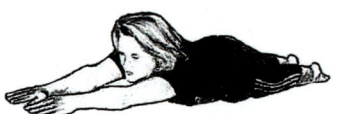

2. **INHALE** as you lift your left arm and leg as high as you can. **EXHALE** them down. **x3**. *Change sides and repeat*

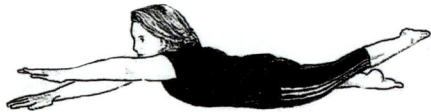

3. Lift your left arm and right leg. Hold and breathe, pushing away on the **EXHALATIONS**. For a variation, you can put your right hand behind your back. Hold for at least **5** breaths.
Change sides and repeat.

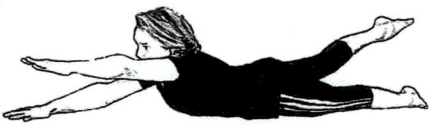

4. **INHALE** as you lift both arms and legs, coming into the **Canoe**.
Hold as in **3**.

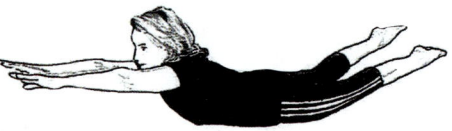

5. Roll over onto your right-hand side with the hands in **Prayer** above your head. Rest the right ear on the upper arm. Arch the abdomen forwards and the feet and hands back so that your body is curved in a banana shape. The back of your right hand and the outside of your foot touch the floor.
Push the fingers away from the toes as in 1.

6. Bring your toes towards your head. Press down with the back of your right hand and the side of your right foot. **INHALE** as you lift your left leg and bring your hand to the knee in the **Side Snake**.
EXHALE them both back to where they were. **x3**
Now pause after the **inhalations** and **exhalations**. Pause for as long as you comfortably can as in **4**, page 91. **x3**

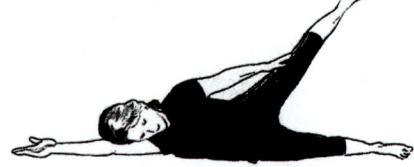

7. Prepare for the **Side Locust**. Bend your right elbow and rest your head on your hand. Place your left palm or fingertips on the floor in front of your waist.
INHALE as you lift both legs. **EXHALE** them down. **x3**

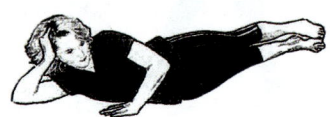

8. Push up on your fingertips and lift the left leg as high as you can. Try and bring the right leg
up to it. Some people find this more comfortable if they curve the legs forwards a little.
Hold and breathe with your mantra.

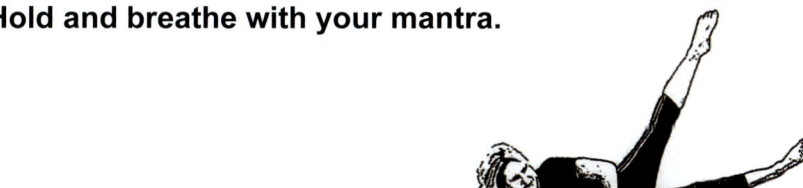

9. Catch hold of your left foot with your left hand. Hold for a few breaths, as in **8**, pulling the leg back on the **exhalations** and stretching the front of the thigh.

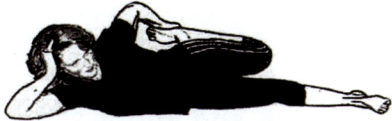

10. Remove the hand from the foot and catch hold of it from the other side of the bent knee. Straighten the leg. You can hold lower down the leg if necessary. Hold as in **8** and **9**, pulling the leg towards the head on the **exhalations**.

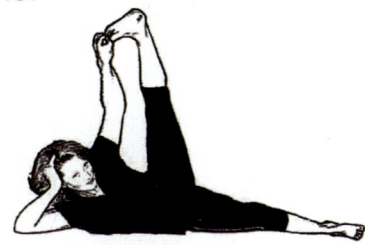

11. Remove the hand from the foot. Roll over onto the abdomen with the hands and feet lifted and wide apart. Hold and breathe for about four breaths in the **Stomach Balance**.

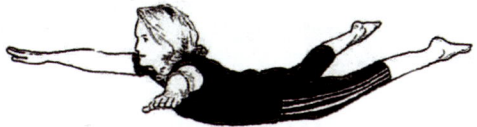

12. Bring the big toes together and swing the hands back into **Flying Bird,** coming into the **Kite**. The chin can be up or down. Squeeze the shoulder blades together and lift the chest as high as you can. With eyes closed, **connect deeply with your mantra** and hold for as long as you can.

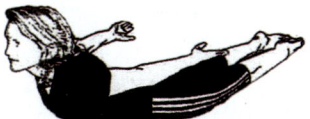

13. When you feel the time is right, make a pillow with your hands. Rest your head on your hands and bring your awareness to your breath. Mentally breathe into the upper back for a few breaths then move down to the waist and lower back in the same way. Imagine you are breathing the vibrations of the mantra into those areas. Feel the expansion and contraction of these three areas when you breathe.
***Return to* 5*. Change sides and repeat*.**

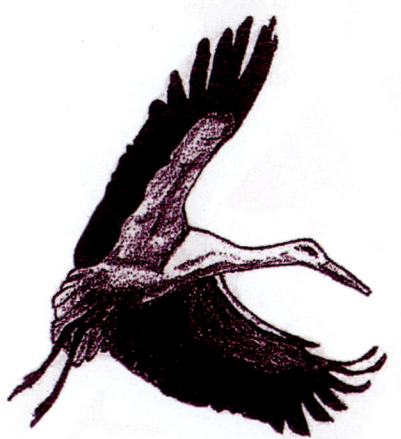

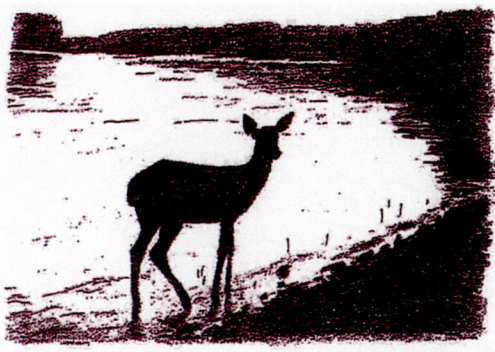

So Hum Class Continued

Continue with your posture work until it is time for the relaxation/meditation at the end of the class. Follow the advice in the second paragraph on page 90 to help you select appropriate postures.

Ideas for the End of the So Hum Class

Deep Relaxation

SO HUM – INHALE and intone the mantra once
EXHALE and intone the mantra twice

Lie on your back. Make sure you are warm and comfortable. Turn the palms downwards. If this feels awkward, move the hands further away from your sides.

Every time you **EXHALE,** allow yourself to sink further and further into the floor. Completely surrender to the floor.
Continue for 5 to 10 breaths.

Now you are going to lift parts of your body as you **INHALE** and **lower** them as you **EXHALE**.

Only lift between **1 and 3 inches** off the floor. We are trying to experience the full weight of the limb or body part. Allow it to feel very relaxed and heavy. When it touches the floor again, allow it to soften and slowly merge into it.

Start with your **right leg**. Lift it slowly as you **INHALE** and lower it slowly as you **EXHALE**.
Repeat 3 or 4 times, feeling the leg getting heavier and heavier.
Change legs and repeat.

Continue with your **right** and **left arm** in the same way.

Now repeat, lifting your legs and arms, but this time, **pause** for a comfortable duration after the **inhalation**. This will increase the feeling of heaviness.

To conclude, repeat the opening **5-10 breaths**, without lifting anything, and feel yourself sinking further and further into the floor.

You can extend this relaxation by lifting the **hips** and the **head** in the same way. I found that, while all my pupils enjoyed and experienced the heaviness when lifting arms and legs, some of them didn't get the same benefits when lifting the hips and head.
To lift the hips, bend your knees a little so that your feet can press into the floor. The feet can be slightly apart. Some experimentation may be necessary.

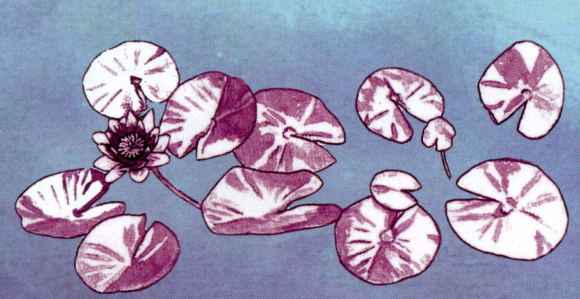
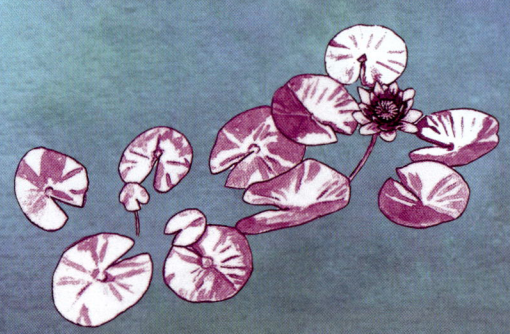

Meditations/Visualisations

These are usually done lying on your back.

You can visualise anything that repeats itself over and over again. The obvious idea is a dripping tap. It drips at regular intervals until somebody turns it off or repairs it.

Method

SO.......**INHALE** as you visualise the drop of water collecting at the end of the tap.

HUM....**EXHALE** as it drips down into the sink below and trickles down the plug hole.

As before, your **exhalations** should be longer than your **inhalations**. Make use of pauses in your breathing to slow down the dripping tap and reinforce your visualisation.

I tried this method after I had made this illustration from photos taken of my friend's antique sink. I found it was much easier with this image in my mind. I showed the illustration to my pupils before they started this meditation and they also found it helpful.

I have blocked out the overflow hole as it made the image too complicated.

Please note this visualisation may not be suitable for someone with prostate cancer.

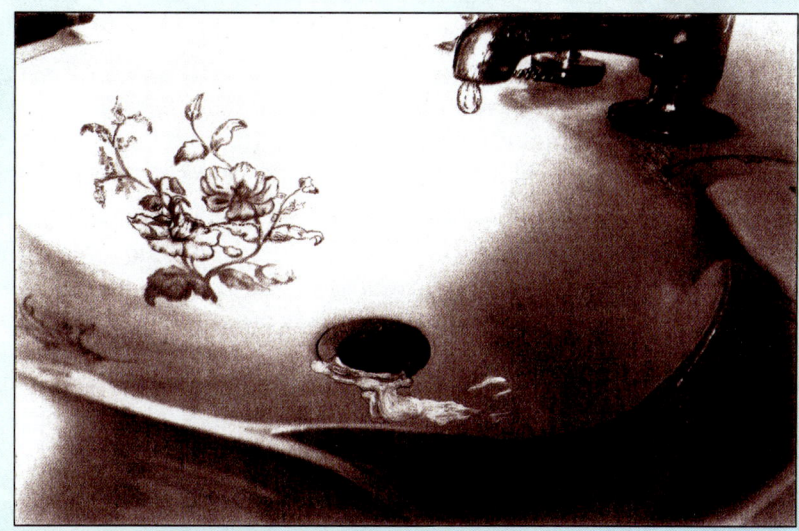

I sometimes use **penguins** to create a visualisation. I have a painting in my shower room of a long line of penguins queuing up on a ledge above a pool of water.

Method

SO........**INHALE** as one penguin comes to the end of the ledge.

HUM.....**EXHALE** as it dives in the water and swims around.

Continue as the next penguin steps up to the end of the ledge. The penguins swim around exploring and catching fish. Eventually they come out of the water one by one.

SO.........**INHALE** as a penguin climbs out of the water onto a bank.

HUM.....**EXHALE** as the penguin waddles over to a bank and sits down.

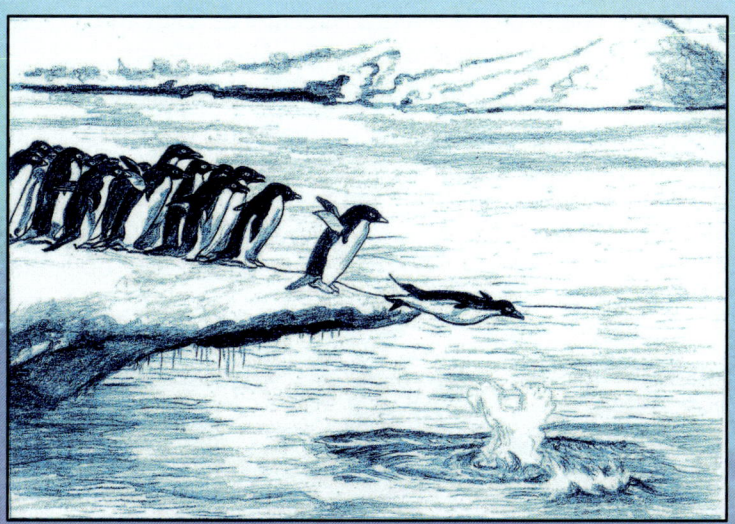

Eventually they all come out of the water and they rest there, warming themselves in the afternoon sun. **Continue repeating the mantra** until you feel it is time to roll over onto your right hand side. **When you are ready**, come to sitting and either finish the class in the usual way or repeat the **So Hum** chant on page 90.

Water Visualisation

Imagine you are water all the way through this visualisation.

Start at the bottom of the Atlantic Ocean, deep down on the dark sea bed, somewhere between England and North America. There are strange deep sea creatures down here with their own lighting systems, and large blue whales. The whales are calling to each other and making weird moaning noises.

A warm current is moving up from the South Atlantic Ocean and you suddenly feel yourself being pushed up towards the surface. Gradually there is more sunlight. The colours become brighter and we see dolphins, large shoals of mackerel and herring and different coloured seaweed.

Eventually we find ourselves bobbing up and down on the surface of the sea, being lulled about by the waves. It is midday and the sun is directly overhead. It is very hot and we soon find ourselves evaporating, turning into mist, and drifting up towards the blue sky. We drift higher and higher until we form part of a fluffy white cloud. A gentle breeze blows us towards the coast of Brazil.

We float above the ocean for several days and nights. Aeroplanes fly overhead and we see large and small boats below. The night sky is very clear. We can see right across the Milky Way and the Crescent Moon gets larger and brighter every night. We see the sun rise to the left. A few glimmers of light flicker over the horizon and then the sun slowly creeps up over the edge of the sea. As it rises, the sky glows with pinks, purples, oranges and yellows. The sun is bright red and orange. The colours are reflected by the sea and when it is half way up over the horizon it looks like a great big ball of fire. Little by little it creeps up over the side of the sea. When it is completely visible the pinks, purples, oranges and yellows streak across the sky for miles and miles in each direction.

As it leaves the sea behind, the sun becomes smaller and the colours fade. By midday it is directly overhead and it is small and shining brightly. Then it moves over to the right side of the sea and exactly the same thing happens again in reverse. Streaks of colour appear in the sky. The sun gets larger and larger and the great big ball of fire slowly disappears over the edge of the sea and the moon and stars shine brightly in the clear night sky.

Then one sunny day we see the coast of Brazil in the distance. At first it is a thin line on the horizon but, as we get closer, it becomes larger and clearer and we can make out the palm trees and beaches and see the little waves lapping on the sea shore. We are floating right over the mouth of the river Amazon. It is three or four miles across as it enters the sea.

The tropical rain forest that it flows through is like a carpet of green stretching out into the distance. The river looks like a shining silver ribbon as it twists and turns through the jungle. We see large towns and ports on the bank at the wide part of the river. Boats sail up and down the river and out into the ocean.

We float over the carpet of green for many days and nights. The silver ribbon below us becomes straighter and narrower as it approaches the mountains of Colombia. There are more spectacular sunrises and sunsets. As we approach the mountains we find ourselves being pushed upwards. We become colder and heavier as we move higher up the side of the mountains. Near the top we condense into drops of rain and fall down heavily onto the rocky slopes below. We find ourselves trickling down little mossy gullies to the stream in the middle of the valley. We merge with the crystal clear mountain stream as it meanders and babbles over the rocky landscape towards the lowland.

As we flow back towards the carpet of green, the stream becomes wider and deeper as other little streams join us. We find ourselves crashing over rapids, large piles of rocks in our path. There is a lot of noise and spray. Then we find ourselves falling over the side of a steep cliff. We become part of a huge waterfall and crash down into a swirling pool of water below. We swirl around in the bottom of the pool and when we reach the surface we are in dense tropical rain forest. It is very noisy. Parrots screech to each other and so do the monkeys as they leap through the trees. The big cats roar loudly. Wild boar and deer come to the side of the pool to drink.

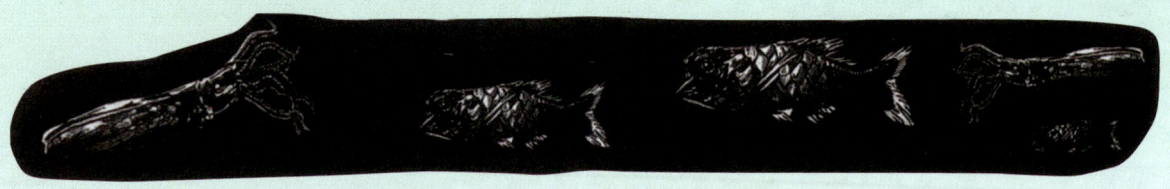

We find ourselves leaving the pool and becoming part of the River Amazon. It is fairly narrow now and the trees meet on top. The monkeys leap above us from one side to the other. As we continue, more rivers join us. As we become wider the trees above part and we see the sun shining brightly overhead. We slow down and become deeper and warmer. Tropical fish, of many different sizes, shapes and colours swim around. Birds stand at the side of the river to catch them. Alligators and all the weird creatures of the tropical rain forest swim in us or come to our banks.

Some of the native indigenous Indians live in clusters of huts close by. They paddle their homemade canoes up and down the river, catching fish and visiting other villages.

As we move further towards the sea, more rivers join us and we start to slow down and form big curves and loops through the forest. Steamy, muddy swamps form at the side of the river. There are more crocodiles and alligators and creepy crawlies.

Further down towards the sea, big towns spring up on our banks and long roads connect them. There is more activity with many boats trading and visiting.

We become wider and wider and deeper and deeper and eventually we taste salt. We have joined the sea and are moving along the sea floor. There are many different coloured seaweeds and fish. We see sharks, dolphins and jelly fish. Sea gulls and albatross swoop overhead. We pass the occasional shipwreck and see large, mysterious indentations in the sea floor.

Then the same warm current that pushed us out of the sea at the beginning of our journey, moves us northwards, back along the sea bed. Sometimes we are pushed higher and we see large shoals of small fish and many dolphins. The ocean changes from light and warm to dark and cold many times until we find ourselves back where we started with the whales and deep sea creatures, at the bottom of the dark sea bed, somewhere between England and North America.

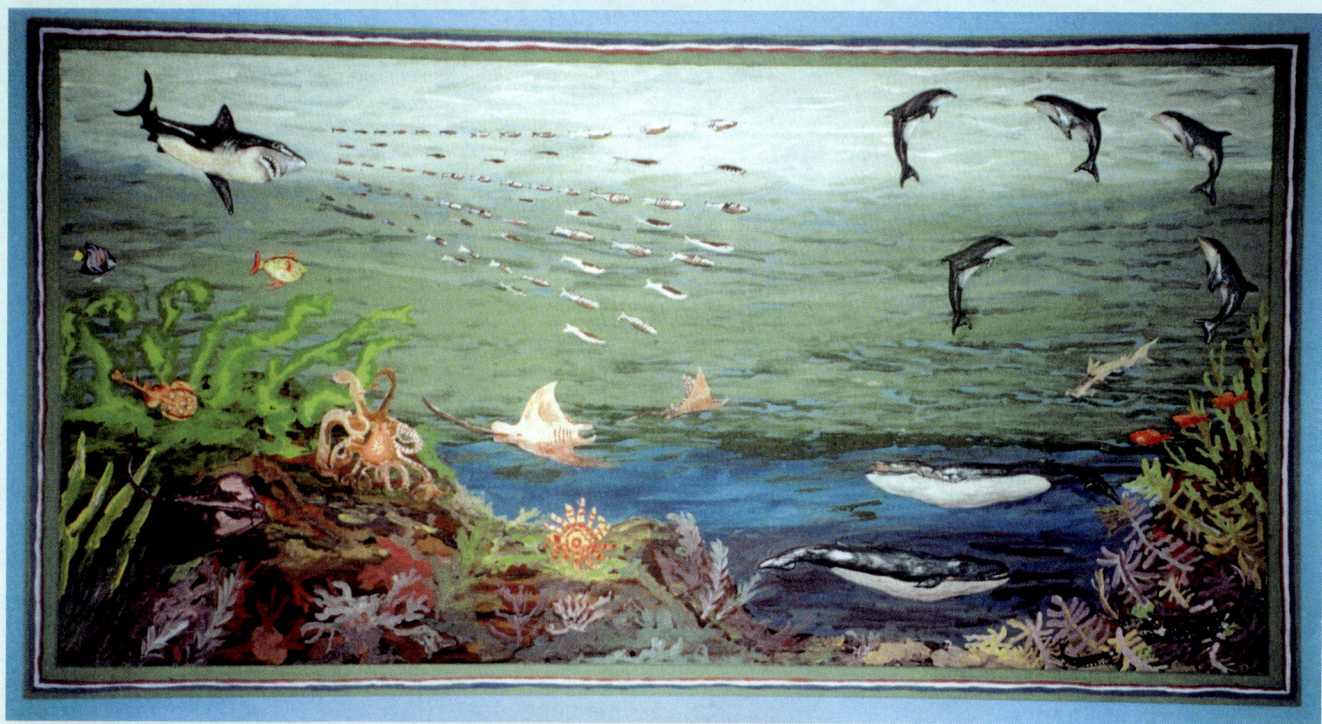

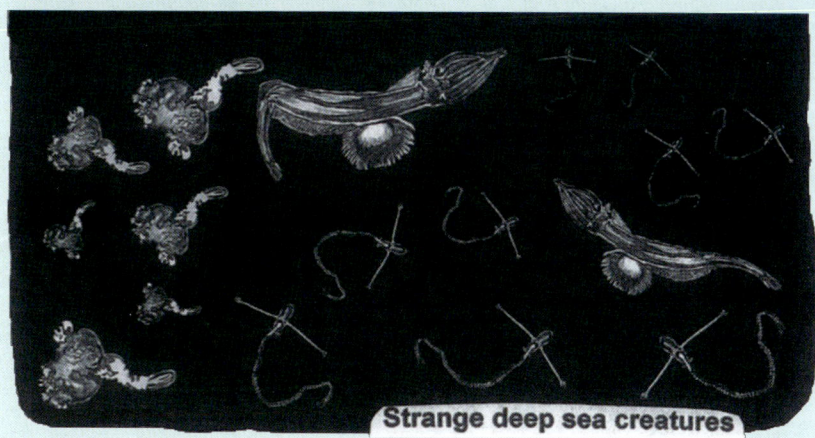

Strange deep sea creatures

I developed this visualisation at about the same time I was working on this large plaque with service users at St. Anne's Opportunity Centre in Newbury. About twelve adults with various disabilities worked on it for about six months. Some staff members also contributed the odd fish or piece of seaweed. It was great fun. The models are made out of plaster. It is 74" by 42".

Practical Ideas for Meditation

In a workshop at the British Wheel of Yoga Congress (BWY), 2008, Swami Krishnapremananda[1], from the Mandala Ashram in Wales, talked about positioning yourself for meditation. He compared it to parking a car. He said you align your car against the pavement and then you walk away from it. When you sit down for meditation, you align the spine and position yourself comfortably and then you can forget about the body and go inwards. I liked this comparison and the idea of having a body-free awareness.

Although some Eastern schools of meditation include uncomfortable practices, such as sitting on your legs so that they go numb (a Chinese lodger told me about this practice), being comfortable is 'the norm'. Here are some suggestions for meditation postures.

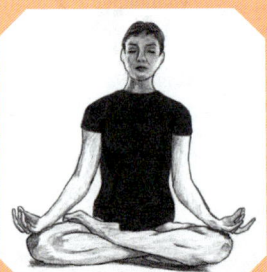

If you are one of the fortunate few who can achieve body free awareness while you sit in **Lotus Pose**, you don't need to read this section.

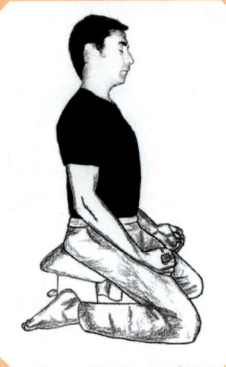

Here is another alternative. Find a comfortable position for your chin. Lengthen the back of your neck to open up the energy channels.

In any posture the same breathing guidelines will apply. **Lift** the **sternum** and make sure the diaphragm and ribcage can move freely. Breathe with a completely relaxed abdomen. Keep the mouth closed unless you are instructed otherwise.

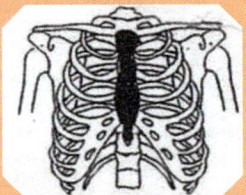

The Sternum

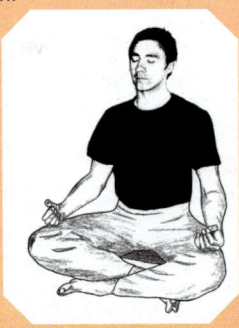

Easy Pose
Rest the feet and legs on something soft. That will prevent you getting 'pins and needles'. Sit on a comfortable amount of blocks and cushions. Sitting with the hips raised is kinder on the lower back.

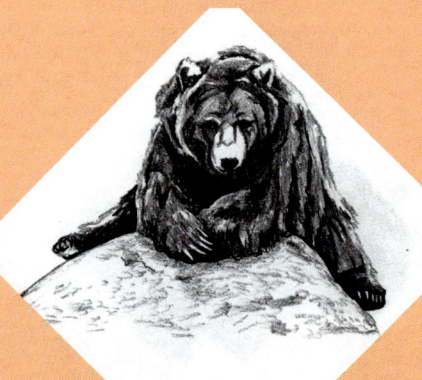

If you are still uncomfortable, find any posture that will allow you to forget about your body, e.g. lying down.

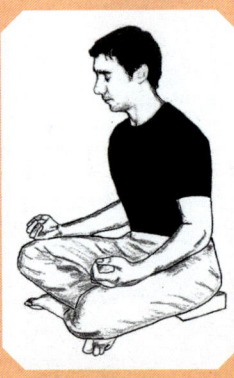

Here the sternum is low and the shoulders have moved forwards. The diaphragm is compressed and its movement restricted. Do not sit like this.

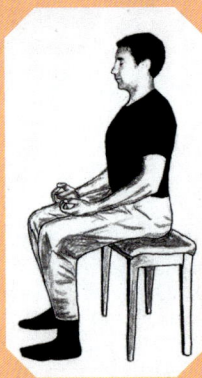

Sit on a chair if you are still preoccupied with your body. Make sure it is the right height and that the seat is comfortable. Energy may escape through cold feet. You may want to keep your socks on.

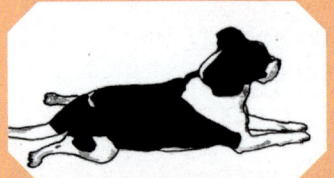

The key words are **relaxed** and **alert**. The most advantageous balance between the **Sympathetic** and **Parasympathetic** Nervous Systems.

Dr. Wayne Dyer said that we live in a house with many different rooms but most of us live in one room the whole time. We push and push to get out of the room...*but the door opens inwards*.

I taught Meditation at Inglewood Health Hydro for five years until it was closed down in 2005. I taught a different group of people for one hour every week and it was a wonderful learning experience. I would like to share some of the insights I gained.

Some people had developed their own way of directing their senses inwards. This often developed in childhood. They hadn't thought of it as meditation and were surprised when I suggested a technique that was similar to their self-discovered method. One man had learnt to slow down his heart beat. Some used visualisation to disconnect from the outside world or to help themselves go to sleep. Some had repeated their names over and over again, like a mantra, to access a different state of consciousness[2].

Among those who were regular meditators, some had had a special, dramatic experience within six months of starting to meditate. Some had tried to repeat the experience and were disappointed because it hadn't happened.

One lady, probably in her forties, who had not meditated before, appeared to access a blissful state during the class. She remained sitting cross legged at the end of the session after having said, 'It's so wonderful, so beautiful'. Regrettably, I left her sitting there. I wish I had waited until she returned to normal awareness and spoken to her about her experience. Maybe she had meditated in a past life and she went back to the point she departed from.

Perhaps it is best to have no expectations when you start to meditate. Just be your wonderful self with unlimited potential and go with the flow.

Out of Body Experiences (OOBEs) were frequently discussed. One young lady felt the separation beginning in the class. It was the first time she had meditated. Another novice meditator told me she had had a prolonged and peaceful OOBE in the other meditation teacher's class at Inglewood. Most people who reported the experience were not disturbed by it but one lady said her husband had stopped meditating because it happened too often.

Following a suggestion from the **Astral Projection Workbook**, by J.H. Brennan[3], I advised that they just wiggle a big toe if they wanted to get back inside their bodies. One lady, a confident OOBE experiencer, said, 'Just wiggle anything'. Here is an interesting quotation from that book:

> *Like Sylvan Maldoon, Monroe believes it is most likely that most - indeed probably all - of us leave our bodies unconsciously during sleep... Muldoon was convinced the etheric moved slightly out of alignment with the physical during sleep in order to absorb the cosmic energy the Hindus call prana and the Chinese call Ch'i. He also believed that almost everyone experienced much fuller projections during sleep.*

I suspect I have had such an experience when I wake up and find my body shaking. After one such shaking experience, a lodger, herself a very experienced astral projector, said, 'Did you have a good night? We went astral travelling together'.

Like most things, a meditation practice can evolve. Some people practise the same way for years and suddenly change. I met a lady who had taught and practised Transcendental Meditation for 14 years and then changed to over-tone chanting. When you have found a particular method that suits you, there will be resistance to change. If you are used to meditating with your eyes closed, it will be disturbing to meditate with your eyes open as is the practice in some schools of meditation, e.g. the Bramachari Women. If you are used to using a mantra, you may find it difficult to concentrate without using one. You may try different techniques but you are likely to return to the method you are familiar and comfortable with.

---

1. Swami Krishnapremananda says it was Swami Anubhavananda, his teacher on the 2007 Vedanta course in India, who first inspired him with this idea.
2. The Victorian poet, Lord Alfred Tennyson said: *A kind of waking trance I have had, quite up from boyhood, when I have been all alone. This has often come upon me through repeating my own name to myself silently till, all at once, out of the intensity of the consciousness of individuality, the individuality itself seemed to dissolve and fade away into boundless being; and this is not a confused state, but the clearest of the clearest, surest of the surest, the weirdest of the weirdest, utterly beyond words, where death was almost a laughable impossibility, the loss of personality (if so it were) seemed no extinction, but only true life.*
3. **The Astral Projection Workbook** by J.H. Brennan, Sterling Publishing. ISBN 0-8069-7306-4

Clearing Your Mind Before Meditation

The emphasis in yoga is always on experimentation and personal verification rather than mere belief. These wise words from George Feuerstein[1] ring particularly true with our meditation practice. The established methods of meditation derive from the experimentation of a teacher or Guru[2] whose ideas or revelations happened to help, inspire and suit other people. If these ideas don't work for you, be pragmatic and **find the car that works**.

Here are some ideas that have been found to help my pupils and others. In some meditation methods, you do not try to stop the thoughts from intruding. You observe them and return to your mantra or chosen point of concentration. These methods aim to create a timeless space for your meditation so that you are less attached to the present moment. In this respect, it is different from **Mindfulness** which emphasises full concentration on the present moment.

As you get older your meditation experience may change. Since turning 70, I find my mind is more nebulous and dreamy. Others in my age group say that their concentration has improved. I always meditate in the morning and my rule is **no breakfast until I have done my meditation**. As I'm pretty dozy in the mornings anyway, I can quite happily sit for a few minutes, just drifting from one thing to the other, without actually meditating.

I found it necessary to separate my meditation from my everyday experience, almost like changing dimensions. My methods have evolved with time. Here are some I have used when necessary.

1. I visualized a black **Delete** button, with the word written in red or white. As my finger pressed the button I thought the word **Delete** very forcefully. The object is to delete everything in your conscious awareness, thus creating a blank space. **After pressing the Delete button**, I inhaled and paused before starting my meditation. Some pupils found this surprisingly effective.

2. I started to take advantage of the hollow, empty, timeless space that you experience during a pause after inhalation and exhalation. If you are not aware of this space, try experimenting. It is best not to completely fill the lungs in the inhalation, just take a normal, complete yogic breath (see page 8) and pause for a comfortable duration. Some people prefer pausing at the end of the exhalation. After you have finished exhaling, your lungs will still be about 20% full of air so you are safe to hold it for some time.

3. I came across two similar ideas. First, when reading **The HeartMath Solution**[3], it introduced a concept called **Freeze-Frame**.

> The term 'freeze-frame' is movie lingo for stopping a film at a single frame to take a closer look…This gives you the power to stop your reaction to the movie at any moment. It lets you take time-out to gain a clearer perspective on what is happening in a single frame…it allows you to tap into a deeper source of intuition and power.'

It then suggests beneficial ways to align your head and heart intelligence. As a prelude to meditation, we are not using it in quite the same way. We are simply **stopping our film** to clear our mind for meditation.

The second similar idea came from a **David Icke** video. I came across my son watching it on his computer. David Icke was suggesting that life is like a DVD. The DVD provides the **information**. When you stop the DVD you **cut off the source of information.**

4. The next idea is more an example of experimentation than one which is likely to appeal to other people.

This method is more dynamic and may seem absurd to some, but it was 'the car that worked' at the time. First I visualised a 'Harry Potter' type wizard holding a magic wand on the right side of my inner vision. The wizard lifted the wand and brought it down to the left and a curtain of gold came across my mind separating my daily experience from my meditation. At the same time, I made a whoosh sound as I exhaled. This reinforced the visualisation. Then I used my breath to keep my mind clear and started to use my mantra.

When I started doing the drawings for **Hanuman's Leap,** I became very involved with the character of Hanuman and substituted him for the wizard. Hanuman sat on the right side of my inner vision holding his golden Mace (see page 53). He lifted it up and swung it down to the left, creating a streak of gold. I made another **whoosh** sound as I **exhaled**, then I paused for as long as I comfortably could and savoured the timeless, hollow, empty space this pause created. Then I started my meditation.

5. You may find it helps to take a few slow, deep breaths, with short pauses to maintain the empty space, before intoning your mantra. On about the third breath, **inhale** fully and then empty the lungs a little so that the breath retention is comfortable, and pause for as long as you can. Return to your mantra, or chosen point of concentration, as you 'top up your inhalation'.

Whenever the outside world starts to intrude, i.e., the thoughts start drifting in, you can recreate the empty spaces during the breath retentions after inhalation and exhalation.

This quotation comes from *Wakening the Global Heart* by Anodea Judith, PH.D., published by Elite Books.

> *As a vehicle of transcendence, meditation is by far the most ancient, tried-and-true, simple, effective, inexpensive, go-anywhere, do-anytime kind of practice there is. It is the vehicle for transcending the mental matrices that keep us behaving in unproductive patterns, beliefs and habits. Meditation allows us to disengage the clutch of life long enough to shift to another gear, a shifting that is desperately needed at this time.*

1. **The Yoga Tradition** by George Feuerstein PH.D. (1998), Published by Hohm Press.
2. **Guru** is a Sanskrit term that connotes someone who is a teacher, guide, expert or master of certain knowledge or field. Some say a Guru leads you from darkness to light.
3. **The HeartMath Solution** by Doc Childre and Howard Martin, (1999). Published by HarperOne.

Nostradamus and Einstein

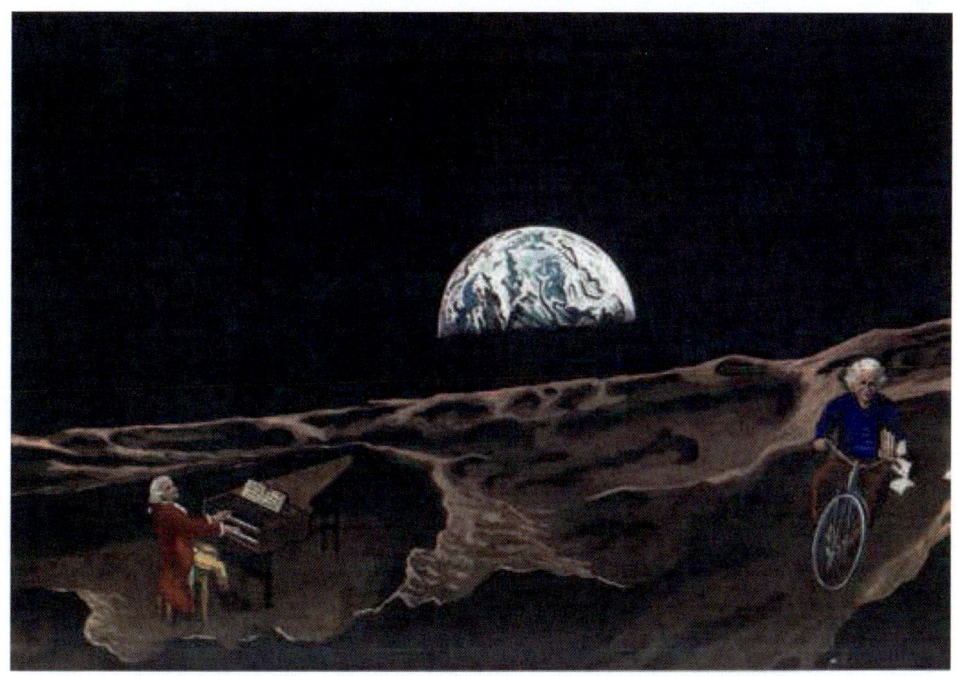

Picture of **Mozart and Einstein on the Moon**, painted by Vani Devi in her 30s

Nostradamus and Albert Einstein were great thinkers who discovered for themselves, how to **take the mind to a point**. I have no doubt many others have achieved this state.

Nostradamus was born in France in 1503. He was an Astrologer and Physician but he became famous for his prophecies. He wrote in four line verses. To access his powers of intuition, he used to stare at a candle flame reflected on a bowl of water.

Albert Einstein (1879 – 1955) was born in Germany. He was a theoretical physicist and is best known for his theories about relativity. He began his famous **thought experiments** (visualising travelling along a beam of light) at the age of 6.

One of his best known quotations is: *We cannot solve problems by using the same kind of thinking we used to create them.*

One method he used to change his way of thinking was to read lots of books and then take a trip on a boat. He would look at the water lapping around, become totally relaxed and wait for the ideas to pop into his head. He had learnt not to try (the effortless state of Yoga Nidra) but to just do his homework and trust and wait.

This is echoed in an experiment I read about in **Spiritual Science of Kria Yoga** by Goswami Kriananda[1].

> *Many years ago, Professor Einstein, along with a number of students, was placed on an electroencephalogram (yes they had them back then) in which the brain wave activity was recorded. The students and Einstein were both induced into a relaxed state as shown by the alpha waves[2]. But, when the students were given a simple problem to solve, the electronic instruments immediately reflected that their minds had moved out of the passive state. However, when Einstein was asked to solve the problem, he was able to remain in a passive state. In short, the students were in a relaxed state; Einstein was in a meditative state.*

A passing comment. If you think I have 'gone over the top' with some of the ideas in this book, you can blame my meditation. Quite a few of the ideas came to me 'out of the blue' when I was meditating.

More Quotations by Albert Einstein

Reality is merely an illusion, albeit a very persistent one.

The only valuable thing is intuition.

All religions, arts and sciences are branches of the same tree.

Science without religion is lame. Religion without science is blind.

The only thing that interferes with my learning is my education.

Few are those who see with their own eyes and feel with their own hearts.

Imagination is more important than knowledge.

---

1. **The Spiritual Science of Kria Yoga** by Goswani Kriananda, 1976. The Temple of Kria Yoga, Chicago.
2. The Alpha state feels like relaxed alertness, with a pleasant feeling of drifting. It is 8 to 12 cycles of electrical activity per second according to most authorities.

Smile, Listen and Pause

Whilst preoccupied with an unresolved problem, I had difficulty steadying my mind during meditation. Thoughts kept intruding and disturbing my concentration. I experimented by combining some of the tried and tested techniques used to quieten the mind. I found a combination that worked for me. My pupils also found it helpful, so I am sharing it with you.

Here is the method in its simplest form:

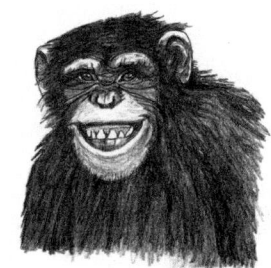

> **Smile** as you **breathe in**
> **Listen** as you **breathe out**
> **Pause** for as long as you comfortably can
> **Continue** in the same way

Explanation

When you smile you stop using words[1].
When you listen intently, you stop breathing and thinking. The mind becomes empty, and hollow and almost timeless. If you ask a group of people to listen to a pin drop, those who concentrate well will stop breathing and thinking.
When you pause after inhalation or exhalation there will be a suspension of mental activities.

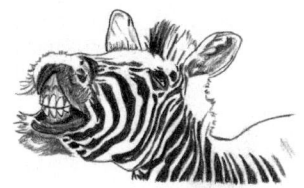

Practical Application

Use the simple method to start with, thinking *Smile, Listen, Pause* as a mantra while you coordinate these actions with the breath. The smile can linger while you exhale. Listen for internal sounds rather than external sounds. When the practice is established you can expand it.

If you use a mantra when you meditate, you can continue using it. When you exhale, listen to it intently. If you have another method of meditating, try combining both methods.

If you have never meditated, try using a one syllable mantra like **Sham** (pronounced Sharm - this is another name for Lord Krishna) or **Aum** (pronounced Om, see page 79). **Repeat** the mantra on the inhalation and exhalation.

Directing concentration to different parts of the body also helps to quieten the mind. You can try **smiling up into the top of your head** on the inhalation. When you pause after the exhalation, your awareness will naturally move down to the abdomen.

When it feels right, **direct your smile to the Heart Centre**. Breathe love and emotional warmth into the middle of the chest. Continue as before, with your awareness in the abdomen during the pause.

Lord Krishna says in the Bhagavad Gita:

> *Whenever the mind wanders, restless and diffuse in its search for satisfaction without, lead it within; train it to rest in the self. Abiding joy comes to those who still the mind. Freeing themselves from the feint of self will, with their consciousness unified, they become one with Brahman.*

Chapter 6, verse 26 and 27. Translation by Eknath Easwaren.
In modern terminology, the last phrase would translate as…*going back to source.*

---

1. After reading the Additional information on the next page, you may conclude that when you smile, your awareness moves to the Heart Brain and that is why words disappear. The Head brain is the only one with words.

Additional information

We need to control the wastage of energy through worrying and over-using the **thinking part** of the brain. The following quotations come from **Energy Balance through the Tao** by Mantak Chia[1].

The head brain is a 'monkey mind', riddled with doubt, shame, guilt and suspicion. It is always thinking, planning and worrying… Scientists have discovered that when people spend a lot of time worrying, their upper (in the head) brain uses a lot of energy. They say the upper brain can use up to 80% of the body's energy, leaving only 20% for the organs. We need to use the brain in the head in order to perform complex functions such as reasoning, making plans and making calculations. These are typical left-brain functions. However, in our daily life of consciousness, awareness and feeling, which is typically governed by the right brain, we can either use the brain in our head or the brain in the gut.

Scientists have recently discovered the same type of neurones found in the 'head brain' in the heart and large and small intestines.

In 1996 an article about the 'hidden brain in the gut' was published in the New York Times. It described the work of researchers who found that the gut, the enteric nervous system[2], functioned similarly to the brain. They had discovered that the large and small intestines had the same type of neurons as are found in the brain and that the gut can send and receive impulses, record experiences, and respond to emotions, in other words, the gut functioned very much like a brain.

If you have already read Heart Opening on page 74 you may be confused. If you combine the above information with that information, it would appear that we have what could be described as three brains.

I put **'brain in heart and gut'** into Google search engine and another world was opened up. If you are still feeling sceptical go to NeuroLogica Blog for a good discussion.

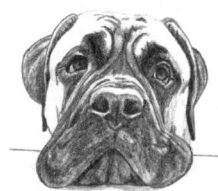

Your facial expression affects the way you feel

In a **Training Magazine** article titled **Coaching the Brains in our Head, Heart, and Gut**[3], I found some lists of associated functions.

The Prime Functions
Our findings indicate that there are three core prime functions for each of the three neural networks, or *brains*:

Heart Brain Prime Functions

Emoting: Emotional processing (e.g., anger, grief, hatred, joy, happiness, etc.)
Values: Processing what's important to you and your priorities (and its relationship to the emotional strength of your aspirations, dreams, desires, etc.)
Relational Affect: Your felt connections with others (e.g., feelings of love/hate/indifference/ compassion/uncaring, like/dislike, etc.)

Gut Brain Prime Functions

Core Identity: A deep and visceral sense of core self and determining at the deepest levels what is *self* versus *non-self*
Self-Preservation: Protection of self, safety, boundaries, hungers and aversions
Mobilisation: Mobility, impulse for action, gutsy courage, and the will to act

Head Brain Prime Functions

Cognitive Perception: Cognition, perception, pattern recognition, etc.
Thinking: Reasoning, abstraction, analysis, synthesis, meta-cognition, etc.
Making Meaning: Semantic processing, language, narrative, metaphor, etc.

The Highest Expressions of each brain are:
Head brain – **Creativity**
Heart brain – **Compassion**
Enteric brain – **Courage**

Mantak Chia says of the smile; *Just by flexing the facial muscles into the position of a genuine smile, we can produce the same effects on the nervous system that naturally go with a natural spontaneous smile. We can actually make ourselves relaxed and happy by taking advantage of this built-in mechanism… Learning to smile down to the abdominal area… is the first step in training the second brain… When the upper brain is resting, brain repair and maintenance occur and new brain cells can grow.*

This quotation comes from Spontaneous Evolution by Bruce Lipton and Steve Bhaerman[4].
Your facial expression actually triggers bodily production of emotional chemistry that is related to both happiness and unhappiness. Emotions specifically shape physiological and physical responses that accompany our behaviours. Conventionally, we tend to perceive that emotions are the driving force behind our behavioural experiences. However, new science has revealed an amazing discovery that our physical expressions can drive emotional responses…Smiling reduces secretion of stress hormones and raises the production of endorphins, which are the body's natural feel-good hormones, while simultaneously enhancing the function of the immune system by increasing T-cell production.

The Pause after Exhalation

The Russian asthma specialist, Buteyko, emphasises the importance of the pause between exhalation and inhalation (Kumbhaka).[5] The blood becomes alkaline when oxygen levels are too high. This causes the symptoms of asthma. The carbon dioxide level in the blood should be 6% to maintain the correct acid/alkaline balance for good health. He says a healthy person should be able to hold the pause after exhalation for 40 seconds. If you can't hold the pause after exhalation for 10 seconds, it is an indication for an asthmatic condition.

These estimates refer to a single breath. As you will be repeating the procedure many times in the **Smile, Listen and Pause** meditation, I suggest a comfortable duration would be about 5 – 12 seconds. It is best not to count as it will interfere with the empty, timeless space you will experience.

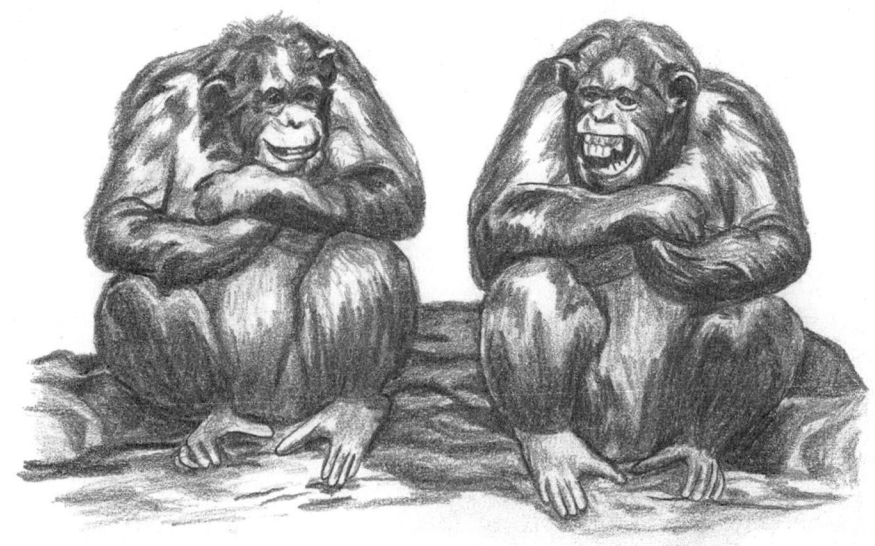

6

1. Published by Destiny Books, 1999.
2. To find out more about the Enteric Nervous System (ENS) go to Wikipedia. It gives reasons why the ENS has been described as the 'second brain'.
3. Their website is: www.trainingmag.com
4. Published by Hay House, 2011
5. 'From an article by Bill Heilbronn in Yoga and Health Magazine titled New Thoughts on Kumbhaka in the light of Buteyko
6. Sketch taken from a photograph taken by Kletr, 'Two chimpanzees having fun.'

Improvising in Meditation

Some Schools of Meditation advise using a mantra you have been given by a Guru for the whole of your life. To depart from it, or disclose it to any body else, would be unacceptable. This method works for many people, for others it is the butt of yogic jokes. Attitudes towards mantras vary greatly as they are used in meditation in many different cultures and circumstances.

Some people like to experiment, others prefer the status quo. Sometimes I simply want to change the inner vibration I am using to accommodate my prevailing mood or inclination.

Influenced by the combined teachings of Sri Sri Ravi Shankar and Dr Wayne Dyer[1], I tried to find a mantra that uses the open **Ah** vowel sound, as in **start**, and closed vowel sound **O**, as in **dog**. I wanted to **INHALE** on the **Ah** and **EXHALE** on the **O**.

I finished up combining the **Sa Ta Na Ma** mantra, as taught by Kundalini Yoga[2], with **Song Kong Tong Dong**. These are four Healing Qigong vibrations.[3]

After experimenting, I developed two different ways to use these mantras in meditation. I use the fingers and thumbs in both as it helps concentration. Due to the creative input, you may find your breathing speeds up and that you have to consciously slow it down at first.

I intuitively used my left hand for the **inhalations** and right on the **exhalations** but you may change the hands around if your intuition tells you it is better that way.

First make yourself familiar with the mantras. Practise the two groups separately until you have memorised them. The best way would be to use the sung version of **Sa Ta Na Ma** on page 89. You can use the same melody for **Song Kong Tong Dong.**

The only rule is: INHALE using a **vibration** from the **Ah** vowel sound mantras and
                                     EXHALE using one from the **Ong** group.

Please note, in this context, **vibration** refers to a syllable.

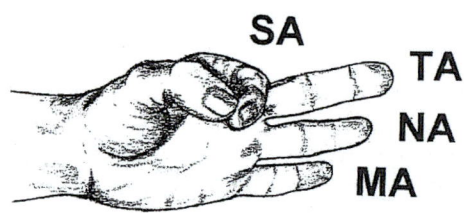
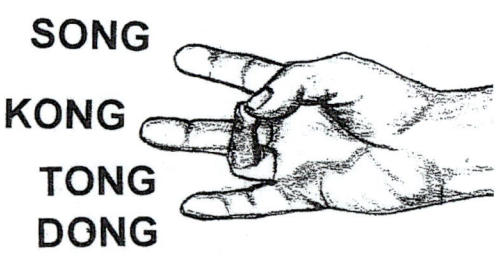

Method 1
I used this method for about four months before the second one evolved.

Stick to the basic rule and use any combinations of the eight vibrations, e.g., **INHALE** to **Sa** (thumb and first finger) and **EXHALE** to **Song** (thumb and first finger of other hand).

Stay there for as many breaths as you want to and then change to another combination. You might move to **Ta** (thumb and second finger) and **Tong** (thumb and third finger).

Stay there for as long as it takes to become involved with the vibrations and then change to another combination. You can repeat one of the vibrations if you want to. You don't use words to decide which vibrations to change to. Let your mind go blank and just observe your mind moving from one to the other when the time is right. It takes a bit of practise. Don't expect your mind to go completely clear at first.

I have been using this method for a few months now. It may evolve further but I am finding it very beneficial at the time of writing. You may decide to skip the first method after you have memorised the mantras and start with this one.

Choose any vibration from the **Ah** group and use the thumb and allocated finger. For example: Use **Ta** with the thumb and second finger touching. This will not change during this particular meditation sitting.

Start with **Song** from the **Ong** group. Use the thumb and first finger of the other hand. Stay with this combination for as many breaths as you choose. When you feel the time is right move on to **Kong**. Change to thumb and second finger. Eventually move on to **Tong** and **Dong** and change to the third and fourth fingers.

To continue, work your way backwards (**Tong   Kong** and **Song**) or return to **Song** and repeat as many times as you want to.

After you have explored this method and worked your way through the other **Ah** vibrations in different meditation sittings, reverse the process. Make one of the **Ong** vibrations your static mantra and change the **Ah** vibrations with their allocated fingers.

Observations
Although you will only be changing one consonant when you move on to the next combination, the vibrations will seem very different. They will change in a subtle way. You will find yourself getting more and more involved with the quality of the vibrations.

You can explore to see if they create different colours and shapes in your mind. I find the **Ah** vibrations are invariably a rusty brown colour in the shape of an archway. My **Ong** vibrations are saucer shaped and have bronze and silver shining from them. Try not to be influenced by what I see. **Open your mind and see what your imagination comes up with.**

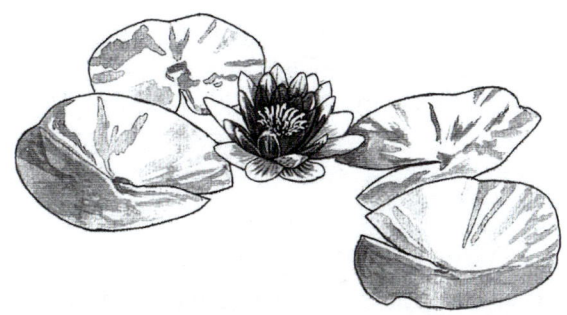

> You may find connecting fingers and thumbs more comfortable if you rest the little fingers on your thighs with the fingers facing downwards.

1. Sri Sri Ravi Shankar, of the Art of Living Movement, asked Dr Wayne Dyer to teach his meditation for Manifestation. One of my pupils gave me Wayne Dyers **Meditations for Manifesting** cassette tapes. They impressed me greatly and I bought his CD with the same title and his book **Manifest your Destiny**. The **Ah** vibration helps you imagine the things you want to happen in your life. He uses the mantra **Om** to help them materialise.

2. This is interpreted by the Kundalini School of Yoga to mean **Existence**, **Birth**, **Death**, and **Rebirth**. In her book, **Kundalini Yoga**, Shakta Kaur Khalsa (Dorling Kindersley, 2010) says …

The thumb and **index** fingers together are for **wisdom**

middle	patience
ring	energy
little	communication

3. I came across this in **The Healing Power of the Breath** (book and CD) by Dr Richard P. Brown and Dr Patricia Gerbarg (Shambhala 2012). (see www.Breath-Body-Mind.com). They talk about the use of **Song Kong Tong Dong** as described by Master Robert Peng. He was taught the art of Healing Qigong by the famous monk Xiao Yao (1889-1985) of the renowned Ch'an Buddhist monastery, Shaolin.

Song	means	**relax**
Kong		**opens divine energy**
Tong		**is to embody divine energy**
Dong		**to understand thoroughly, to be insightful and to see clearly**

Please note that although it is interesting to know the meaning/interpretation of a mantra, when you are meditating there should be no words in your mind to construct a meaning, so it becomes irrelevant.

Standing Visualisation/Meditation

This evolved at the British Wheel of Yoga Congress, 2014. In a workshop with Aki Omori[1], we were taught to imagine we were a Zygote (see The Method below and images on the next page and Additional Information). We drifted around the room in this imaginary state for about twenty minutes.

Later, I went on an outdoor meditation with Muriel Goss. We stood down by the lake in the beautiful Warwick University campus while Muriel suggested various sensations we could concentrate on. As we were standing there in the company of Chinese geese, wild birds and ducks, I realised that we are still living in a zygote-like bubble. We are not aware of it because our limited five senses do not pick up the information. Our senses detect what is needed for our survival. More information could overload our awareness and cause complications. However, a few very special people do have extra-sensory perception and they can see it. They are sometimes called **seers**.

Scientific instruments can now detect this bubble. If you put 'the human aura and energy field' into your browser's search engine, another dimension will unfold. The photography of Harry Oldfield is another area to explore.

Before you start this Visualisation/Meditation, study the images and the information about them on the next page and read the **Additional Information**.

The Method

Stage 1
As soon as an egg is fertilised, its electrical charge changes from negative to positive. This prevents further penetration. After a human egg is fertilized, it takes between 24 and 36 hours to divide into two identical cells. Each cell contains the chromosomes from the mother and father, 23 from each. This is called a **zygote**. It stays like this for 12 hours before each cell divides, creating four smaller identical cells. By the third day there are 16 identical cells.

We are going to imagine we are a two-celled zygote. Each one of us has been in this state for about 12 hours of our existence. In these two cells are all the information and potential to create the highly complicated, miraculous beings we are today.

From a standing position, with your arms floating out to your sides, feel that your body is the connecting layer between two cells. There is a cell behind and a cell in front. You are enclosed in an egg sack and nourished by the egg yolk. You don't have a top or a bottom. You will not be connected to anything until you become imbedded in the womb lining in about five days. By this time, the cells will start to differentiate and behave in different ways.

Start to move around very slowly, imagining your body is in the middle of a large balloon with your whole potential in front of you and behind you. You are floating about in a warm, comfortable environment. A zygote can't see, hear or think and doesn't even know it exists. It responds to gravity so will make contact with the lining of the fallopian tube sometimes while remaining separate and moving on. It is pushed to its destination by small hairs on the tube lining.

While pretending to be one, you will obviously need to open your eyes to avoid collisions. Drift around in this state of non-experiencing potential for a few minutes. At an appropriate time, rediscover yourself as the conscious, feeling, loving, thinking and creative human entity that you are today.

Stage 2
Having moved into the present reality, remain standing and become aware that you are still in a balloon of energy but you can only see and experience the material layer in the middle which is your body. This balloon is made up of different types of energy; some of these are illustrated and explained on the next page.

Imagine you are back in the balloon with all these complex energies surrounding your body from the front, back and sides. **This time you are a conscious, feeling and thinking being**. Move around slowly as before. If you are in a class your energies will overlap.

Drift and intermingle for an appropriate length of time before returning to normal awareness.

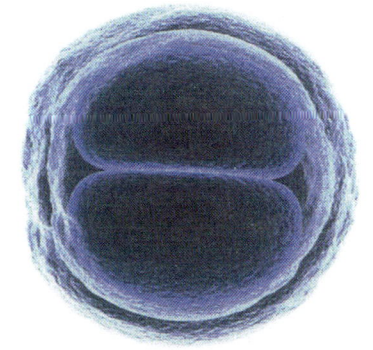

1

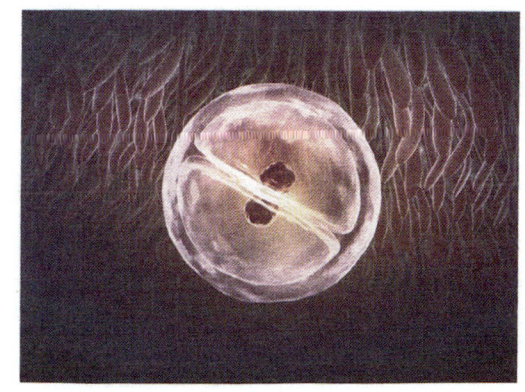

2

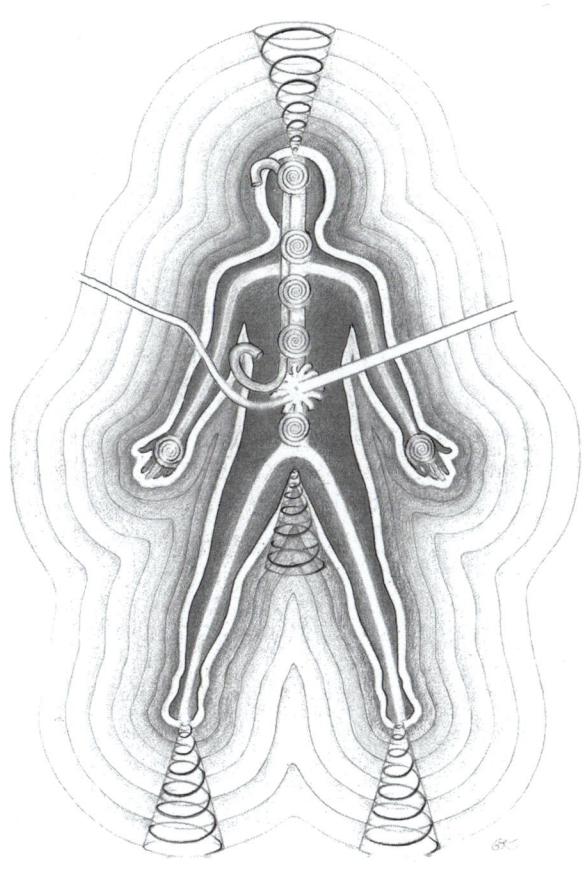

3

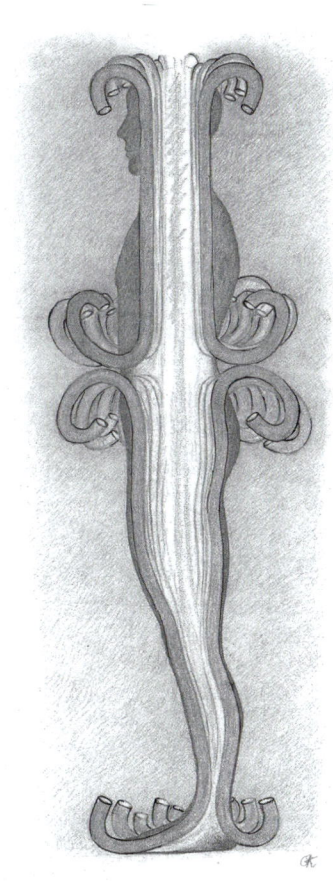

4

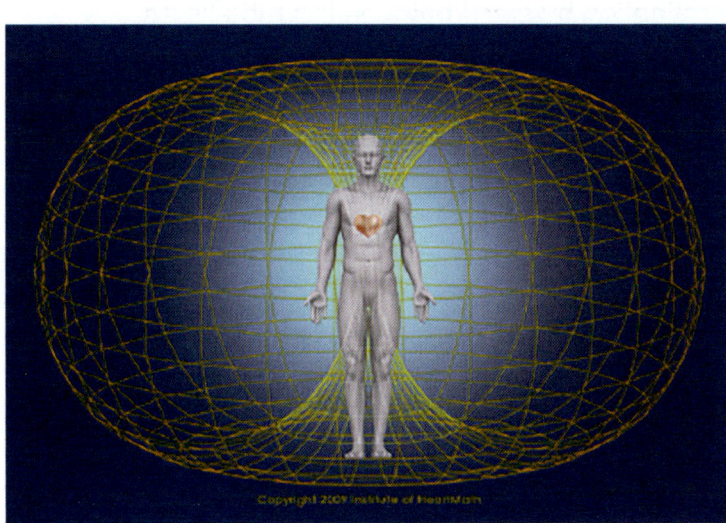

5

1. is a two-celled zygote.
2. is a zygote being pushed along the fallopian tube by tiny hairs.
3. is the **Energy System Complete – Front view**.
4. is the **Tubes Complex – Side view**.
5. The Heart's Electromagnetic Field used with permission from the HeartMath Institute. © 2017 HeartMath Institute.

Information about the Illustrations

3 and **4** are from **Energetic Anatomy** by Mark Rich[2]. When he was a child, Mark saw different types of energy coming from people. He thought everybody else could see them as well. When he described what he saw to a nun at school she reacted in a disapproving way. He thought he would finish up in Hell and even self-harmed to stop himself seeing the shapes and colours.

When he was older he took up Martial Arts and started to 'see energy' again. His book is the result of his re-discovered gift. The two drawings from his book are by Gosha Karpowicz, a yoga teacher and artist. She gave me permission to include them. She told me that it took a long time to get them the way Mark Rich wanted them to be. They had to revise them many times until they represented accurately what he saw.

5. This quotation comes from **Living in the Heart** by Drunvalo Melchizedek[3]. It describes the shape of the electromagnetic field we create.
Scientists have proved that the human heart generates the largest and most powerful energy field of any organ in the body, including the brain in the skull. This electromagnetic field is about 8 – 10 feet[3] in diameter, with the axis centred in the heart. Its shape resembles the donut form of the torus, which is often considered the most unique and primal shape in the universe.

1. Titled **Front body, Middle Body, Back Body - Yoga through Embryology.**
2. **Energetic Anatomy,** published by Wave of the Future, Inc., 2004.
3. **Living in the Heart,** Light Technology Publishing, 2003. Please note that scientific instruments now pick up a much wider field than 8-10 feet.

Additional Information

There are different definitions of a **zygote**. Some sources say that a zygote is a first single fertilised cell. Others say it is that cell and the one that divides into two. The information I have used here comes from **The Human Body Book**, by Steve Parker, published by Dorling Kindersley Limited, 2007.

As we will not be using words when we are imagining our first few hours on this planet, it doesn't really matter what we are called. The important concept is that each one of us has been a two-celled miracle of potential for 12 hours of our existence.

Here are a few quotations that are relevant to this visualisation/meditation. They convey the way ancient yogis thought about the human body and the subtle energy system.

In Nathamuni's **Yoga Rahasya**[1] we read (Sloka 4-22): *The body comprises nadis, flesh, junctions of nadis, organs, joints, bones and tubes. These are different colours and shapes, and some are all over the body, while others are localized.*

Nathamuni lived in the 9th century. It was known that he had written this text but it was lost. When Krishnamacharya (a direct descendent of Nathamuni) was 16 years old he went to a particular tamarind tree on the banks of the River Tamraparani, where the yogis of old used to sit. He went to a nearby holy shrine and, following the instructions of an old man, eventually had the whole manuscript transmitted telepathically to him. He could remember it very clearly. It was eventually translated by his son T.K.V. Desikachar. It was published in 1998 by Krishnamacharya Yoga Mandiram, ISBN 81-87847-19-0

In **Tantrik Yoga**[2] by J. Marques Riviere we read: *The nadi is not simple. It is made of subtle matter, composed of various forces…The yogis who have described these nadis to me have spoken of them as 'tubes', luminous arteries, have spoken of magnificent and changing colour, which varies according to the power and quality of the prana circulating through them. The texts describe them as 'fine as the threads of a spider's web'. Also from the same source: In the Indian Maya tradition… there are curious details of the 'air tubes' along the spine, which incontestably correspond to the Hindu nadis.*

Drunvalo Melchizedek tells us about yet another energy body in **Living in the Heart**, see above.

The human lightbody that surrounds the body for about fifty-five to sixty feet in diameter,
the **Mer-Ka-Ba***, has a secret inherently connected to the sacred space of the heart.*

1. Published in 1998 by Krishnamachara Yoga mandiram, ISBN 81-87847-19-0
2. **Tantrik Yoga**, spelt with a k instead of the usual c, was published in 1970 by Rider and Co and Samuel Weiser. ISBN 877728-006-**1**

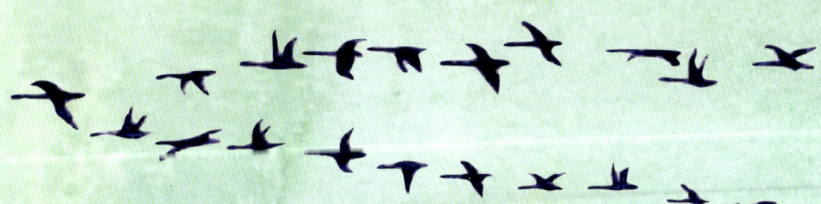

The Inner Sound

I first wrote about this in **Yoga Expanded and Simplified** in 2009. I am revising it here.
I became interested in the **Inner Sound** when I heard that some Buddhist monks use it during meditation. Somebody directed me to a website in 2001, before I had learnt how to use a computer. It clearly demonstrated the potential of this electronic-sounding noise. You can still reach this site by entering: **Find the Inner Sound PcE-Training,SEZ**. I could not download their sound recording but you can hear a similar sound on my website www.koolkatpublications.co.uk

I am referring to the high-pitched electronic sound you might hear when you put your head on the pillow at night and it is dark and quiet. Some people are very familiar with this sound, others can train themselves to hear it and some don't hear it at all.

I always mentioned the inner sound when I taught meditation at Inglewood Health Hydro, to a different group of people, every week for five years. Some had confused it with Tinnitus. It is quite different. Often someone would say they had been disturbed by the noise and had gone to their doctor about it. One said a Buddhist monk had eventually explained it to her. Most had been troubled by it when they were going through a stressful time. I came to the conclusion that one of the functions of the noise was to distract people from their problems. Suggested making friends with the noise and using it to find relief from what was upsetting them.

I recently came across this quotation when I looked up **Nada Yoga** on Wikipedia. It is from the Surangama Sutra, a text of the Chan school of Chinese Buddhism.

How sweetly mysterious is the Transcendental Sound of Avalokiteshvara! It is pure Brahman Sound. It is the subdued murmur of the seatide setting inward. Its mysterious Sound brings liberation and peace to all sentient beings who in their distress are calling for aid; it brings a sense of permanency to those who are truly seeking the attainment of Nirvana's Peace…

I was unable to find any recent research into this sound so here is some information from the **PcE-Training,SEZ** website quoted above.

It was a constant companion in the womb while we waited several months to be born. It reminds us of deep comfort and rest.

*Under normal circumstances, we pick it up when the brain is charged with high energy and the body is completely relaxed. If you listen carefully you can hear a mixture of sounds. It is in the **7 to 9 kHz range**…*

It is comparable to the chirping sound of a cricket or the sound of an electrical motor running at high speed…

How the sound originates is still very unclear. One thing we know is that the sound is perceived in the centre of the temple bones[1] and it is also generated there…

The last quotation would explain why we might pick up the sound when we do the meditation in the **So Hum** sequence (**5** on page **91**). When we concentrate on the front of the top of our head we tend to pick it up. It is likely to be the electrical sound from all the organs in the body. They are in constant communication with the brain in the head.

Some people say that when we tune into our **inner sound** we are also tuning into the heart beat of our planet. This is because planet Earth is a big magnet which creates an electrical pulse. This is in the same frequency range that I have mentioned above.

A friend, who was troubled by his psychic abilities in about the 1970s, spoke to a psychiatrist about the **inner sound**. He described it as two alternating pitches of sound that were similar to the very high **F** and **G** or **F sharp** or **G sharp**, about 3½ octaves above middle C.

---

1. The recognition of sounds, their tones and loudness, takes place in the **temporal lobes**.

Glossary

Advaita Vedanta. The creator and the created are considered one and the same. Matter is energy vibrating at different frequencies. This echoes Einstein's equation, $E=MC^2$, meaning energy =matter. The different dimensions and spiritual landscapes are energy functioning in different ways. In some philosophies and religions, the creator and created are two separate entities.

Ashram. Usually a secluded residence of a spiritual community with teachers, and often based around a particular Guru.

Bhagavad Gita. This is a dialogue between Lord Krishna and Arjuna, from about 2,000BC. It was transmitted orally for many generations and finally narrated by Vyasa in about 550BC.

Hatha Yoga. This is one of the four paths of yoga as described by Lord Krishna in the Bhagavad Gita. Hatha Yoga develops the full potential of the body and mind through systematic practices. These include Asana, posture work to keep the body fit and connected to the brain, Pranayama, to utilise the vast energy potential in the human being, and meditation, to utilize the full potential of the mind.

Hatha Yoga Pradipika. This is a classic Sanskrit manual, written by Swami Svatmarama in about 15th century AD. It is derived from old Sanskrit texts and his own experiences. It advises the aspiring yogi on how to develop an intense spiritual practice.

Heart Centre. The area associated with love and compassion in the middle of the chest.

Kundalini. This is usually depicted as a powerful energy coiled like a snake or serpent at the base of the spine. Awakening the kundalini can be spontaneous or controlled. There are many different experiences associated with it, e.g., in Tantric Yoga it can have sexual connotations. In the Hatha Yoga Pradipika it is a disciplined controlled awakening brought about through many hours of Pranayama.

Mantra. This is a verbal vibration, or resonance, that has a beneficial effect on the body and mind. It can be spoken, sung or thought. It can be one or more syllables, a phrase, a sentence or many sentences. The Hail Mary in the Roman Catholic Church is a long mantra but there are longer ones in the Jewish canticles. A mantra is repeated many times and used as a point of concentration to steady the mind. People can make up their own mantras, and sometimes a particular word takes over a persons mind and it appears that a mantra has been given to them.

Maya. This is the rope that binds man to the illusory world. It is the power which makes form appear real.

Pranayama. **Prana** means **life force** and **ayama** means **control** or **mastering**. It involves many different methods of breathing. When these are combined with other techniques, such as the **Bandhas**, our energy potential can be developed.

Pratyahara. Withdrawing the five senses away from the outside world and directing them inwards.

Samakaras. Deep mental impressions produced by past experiences. They can be dormant impressions from our past lives.

Sanskrit. This was the language of the ancient civilisation which developed on the banks of the Indus River in what is now Pakistan. We find the earliest evidence of yoga there.

Throat Centre. This is the Vishuddha Chakra in the throat. It acts as a bridge between the higher and lower intelligence in the body. What is felt there will be a reflection of the relationship between the abdomen, heart and brain in the head.

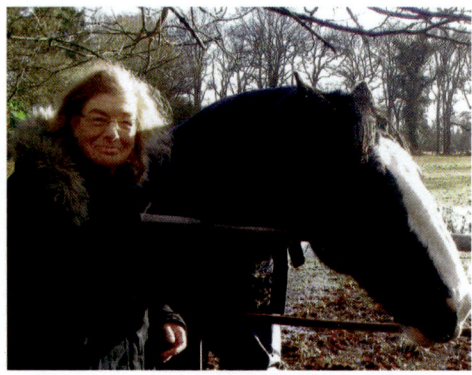

Salutations from the Author

May your yoga bring you joy and contentment.

*Love and Light and rivers of OM
from*

Vani Devi